Joannie
Happy Birthday.
Much love
Paul, Wendy, & Richard

The Perfect Gentleman

THE Perfect Gentleman

The remarkable life of Dr James Miranda Barry, the woman who served as an officer in the British Army from 1813 to 1859

June Rose

HUTCHINSON OF LONDON

Hutchinson & Co (Publishers) Ltd
3 Fitzroy Square, London W1

London Melbourne Sydney Auckland
Wellington Johannesburg and agencies
throughout the world

First published 1977

Set in Monotype Imprint

Printed in Great Britain by The Anchor Press Ltd
and bound by Wm Brendon & Son Ltd, both of
Tiptree, Essex

ISBN 0 09 126840 0

'That an Habit of Secrecie is both Politicke and Morall.'
'Of Simulation and Dissimulation.'

Bacon's *Essays*

Contents

List of Illustrations

Between pages 48 *and* 49

Prologue

War office: Selected Personal Files: WO:138:1830
This class at present consists of one file relating to Dr James Barry, M.D.

25 Duke Street,
Westminster
July 25, 1865

Inspector General
Dr James Barry
Address
14 Margaret Street
Cavendish Square

Disease 'Diarrhoea'

Sir,
I have the honor
to report that the Officer,
named in the margin
died at 4 o'clock
AM this morning
I have the honor to be,
Sir,
Your most obedient humble
servant
D. R. McKinnon M.B.,
S. Surgeon Major

There was nothing remarkable about the death certificate.

The following day, Dr Barry's death was duly registered in the District of All Souls in the County of Middlesex. A senior Inspector General of Hospitals in Victoria's Army was dead and the correct procedure had been adopted. On this form Dr Barry's age (about seventy) and sex (male) were entered.

It was witnessed with the mark of an X by Sophia Bishop, the Irish charwoman who laid out the body.

If Sophia Bishop had kept silent about what she discovered on the death-bed, the scandal would never have spread. But she was outraged, stunned. 'The devil, a General,' she said, in words that echo down the years. 'It's a woman. And a woman that has had a child.'

It was 1865 – the year the 'first' woman doctor in Great Britain, Elizabeth Garrett Anderson, graduated. And yet another woman – James Barry – had already served with distinction as physician and surgeon for forty-six years in the British Army. She had risen from Hospital Assistant to Inspector General, second only to the Director General in the Medical Department, and she had died as an officer – and a gentleman.

On the face of it, it was scandalous – unbelievable. For two weeks no word of the story reached the public. But in the new London clubs on St James's and Pall Mall, in the pot houses and the gin shops, tongues wagged and the gossip grew.

By the 14th of August *Saunders News Letter*, a Dublin paper, broke the story of 'A female army combatant'. The *Manchester Guardian* reprinted the article a week later, and the *Whitehaven News*, a Cumberland paper, picked up the scandal on the 24th of August. Rumour had flown so far that the authorities could no longer afford to ignore it. The Registrar General of Somerset House felt bound to ask Staff Surgeon Major McKinnon a delicate question:

It has been stated to me that Inspector-General Dr James Barry who died at 14, Margaret Street on the 25th July, 1865 was, after his death found to be a Female.

As you furnished the Certificate as to the cause of his death, I take the liberty of asking you whether what I have heard is true, and whether you yourself ascertained that he was a woman and apparently had been a mother?

Perhaps you may decline answering these questions: but I ask them not for publication but for my own information.

I have the honor to be Sir
Your faithful Servant
George Graham
Registrar General

It was an astonishing question to put to a Staff Surgeon in the Recruiting Department of the British Army. The penny post of those days was rapid and reliable and the following morning Staff Surgeon McKinnon penned his reply.

I had been intimately acquainted with that gentleman for a good many years both in the West Indies and in England and I never had any suspicion that Dr Barry was a female.

I attended him during his last illness and for months previously for bronchitis and the affection causing his death was diarrhoea, produced apparently by errors in diet.

On one occasion after Dr Barry's death, I was sent for to the office of Sir Charles McGregor (Army Agents) and there the woman who performed the last offices for Dr Barry was waiting to speak to me.

She wished to obtain some perquisites of her employment which the Lady who kept the lodging house in which Dr Barry had died had refused to give her.

Amongst other things she said Dr Barry was a female and that I was a pretty doctor not to know this and that she would not like to be attended by me. I informed her that it was none of my business whether Dr Barry was a male or a female and that I thought that he might be neither, viz. an imperfectly developed man.

*She then said that she had examined the body and it was a perfect female and that there were marks of her having had a child when very young. I enquired: how have you formed that conclusion? The woman, pointing to the lower part of her stomach said 'From marks here' (*striae gravidarum – *the 'stretch marks'). 'I am a married woman and the mother of nine children and I ought to know.'*

The woman seemed to think that she had become acquainted with a great secret and wished to be paid for keeping it.

I informed her that all Dr Barry's relatives were dead, and that it was no secret of mine, and that my own impression was that Dr Barry was a hermaphrodite.

But whether Dr Barry was male, female or hermaphrodite I do not know . . .

Staff Surgeon McKinnon added that as he could swear to the

identity of the body as being a person whom he had known for eight or nine years, he himself had 'no purpose in making the discovery . . .' An amazing admission, explicable only in terms of McKinnon's loyalty to a fellow officer who had shown a profound distaste for physical examination throughout a long career.

For the Army, the aristocratic Army, it was a highly embarrassing and contentious story. Despite the persistent rumours and the gossip, the staff at the Horse Guards did *not* see fit to order a post-mortem.

Not only Dr Barry but many other victims succumbed to the outbreak of diarrhoea during that hot summer of 1865. In the wealthy parish of Marylebone 300 people died in the first week of July. Open cesspools and streets with 'houses so dirty and dilapidated that the heart sickens at the sight of them' spread the outbreak, which proved 'unusually fatal'. No doubt the Army fervently hoped that the talk, like the heat, would soon subside.

But a few days later the *Medical Times and Gazette* (medicine's most respectable journal) took up the story. From *Saunders News Letter*, the *Medical Times* reprinted information about the incident 'so extraordinary that were not its truth capable of being vouched for by official authority, the narration would certainly be deemed absolutely incredible . . .'

To the *Saunders* story, the *Medical Times* added its own, somewhat sanctimonious, rider.

The above has been the subject of not a little 'club tattle'. There need be no hesitation . . . in our stating what we have heard. The author has fallen into many inaccuracies but he is correct in the main point – the sex of the deceased. The deceased was very well known and many were the stories and surmises circulated during his (?) lifetime . . . the physique, the absence of hair, the voice, all pointed one way and the petulance of temper, the unreasoning impulsiveness, the fondness for pets were in the same direction.

Their concluding remarks were significant. They referred to Sophia Bishop and her discovery of Dr Barry's sex. 'About this point she [Sophia] was very positive indeed . . . Moreover she asserted, with equal assurance and decision, that there were undoubted signs of maternity. In these conclusions the woman was supported and corroborated by others.'

The *Medical Times* it seems was privy to part, at least, of the 'inside story'. The names of the others who corroborated Sophia Bishop's story have never emerged. But there were plenty to deny it.

The Deputy Inspector of Hospitals, Edward Bradford, wrote disdainfully to the *Medical Times*:

The stories which have circulated since his [*Barry's*] *death are too absurd to require serious refutation. There could not have been any doubt among people who knew him, on the subject of his physical constitution which was really that he was a male in whom the development of the organs of sex had been arrested from the sixth month of pregnancy. It is sad that no qualified persons took the opportunity of his death to examine closely the physical condition of the deceased . . .*

Like Staff Surgeon McKinnon, Deputy Inspector Bradford did not really know the sex of Dr Barry. His letter amounted to a military splutter.

Across the Channel in Paris an army magazine was wondering whether Inspector Bradford had 'some reason to wish to stop public curiosity regarding his ex-colleague . . .' Whatever else Deputy Inspector Bradford achieved, it was *not* a reduction in public curiosity regarding Dr Barry. Nearly fifty years later, when moving office, the Army Agents and Bankers, Sir Charles McGregor, who offered a financial service to individual officers as well as to Army Units, came across mementoes of her. A letter they wrote in June 1914 to Colonel Johnstone of the Royal Army Medical Corps, suggests that they, at any rate, had little doubt of Barry's sex:

In going through a number of the papers, we have come on the enclosed which, incidentally, is a draft of two memoranda of the late Dr James Barry. It gives some particulars of his service and is, I believe, in 'his?' own handwriting. I also send you one of his (?) cards and a commission which you may care to have as a memento of an extraordinary woman . . .

The Army Agents took charge of Dr Barry's affairs after death. They knew more than anyone else about the estate, so that their comment on the 'extraordinary woman' must be regarded as important evidence.

The doctor lies buried in Kensal Green Cemetery. The grave now lies derelict and overgrown, the headstone flattened to the the ground, the wording almost indecipherable. It was originally in a prominent position. Only by consulting a dusty old volume of burial records and studying a plan of the graveyard can one locate the plot where Dr Barry lies. The inscription on the sandstone slab, broken and almost indecipherable, simply says:

DR JAMES BARRY
INSPECTOR GENERAL
OF ARMY HOSPITALS
DIED 15TH JULY 1865
AGED 71 YEARS

Dr Barry in fact died on the 25th of July. But then so much of the doctor's *life* is inaccurately recorded that it is hardly surprising that even the date of her death is wrong.

In the controversy that still persists about her sex, the extraordinary achievements of Inspector General James Barry as doctor, surgeon and social reformer remain overshadowed. Too many scandalous questions remain unsettled.

Who was she? How did she manage to conceal her sex from the Army for forty-six years? Why did she decide to take on a man's role and a man's work?

What is undeniable is that from 1813 to 1859 she became an outstanding Army Surgeon and a physician who practised preventive medicine years ahead of her time. The ordinary soldier and the outcasts of society in the Colonies where she served had reason to remember her with gratitude. Yet only in South Africa is her name remembered. For over a hundred years controversy has obscured the significance of her extraordinary adventure.

I

'Known by Lord Buchan, nephew of Mr B'

No family came forward to claim James Barry when she died. Despite the scandal of her sex and the efforts of biographers to solve the mystery for the past hundred years it has proved impossible to establish her identity with absolute certainty. Perhaps that was her intention.

Certainly she appears to have been deliberately vague about her birth, even in official army documents. 'About 1799' is the date she gives, while stating to the day the details of her postings around the world during forty-six years of army service. The ambiguity of her birthdate – and in the original even the words themselves are smudged – seems curious, almost as if she chose to be known only by her public persona. And since she was born many years before the compulsory registration of births, her parents' names and circumstances may be lost for ever.

Early biographers claimed the most extravagant origins for her. She is variously represented as the illegitimate daughter of the Prince Regent, the bastard child of the Duke of York or of Lord 'Hellgate' Barrymore, and the legitimate grand-daughter of a Scottish Earl, almost certainly Lord Buchan. Nobody doubted that she was high-born, but her only known relative was, in fact, definitely plebeian. 'Known by Lord Buchan, nephew of Mr B, painter' states a note beside her name in an Edinburgh University Class Register of 1810, testifying to her connection with James Barry, R.A., one of the most notable – and notorious – history painters of the eighteenth century. 'A little, shabby, pockmarked man in a dirty old coat with a scarecrow wig, living for the most part on bread and apples' was how his contemporaries saw him, but despite his perpetual poverty and his savage temper James Barry had a wide and distinguished circle of friends. He supped regularly at the Essex Head in the Strand with Dr Johnson, Garrick, Sheridan and other members of their circle, and enjoyed the patronage of a fellow Irishman, Edmund Burke, at whose expense he travelled to Europe to study the great masters of the past. Artists, politicians and even aristocrats liked to drink porter at his untidy studio in Soho; despite his loud voice and crude manners Dr Barry's 'uncle' was welcomed in the drawing-rooms of the blue-stockings, those literary women 'professing a philosophic mind, intent on matters higher than their toilet'.

Foremost among his friends was General Francisco de Miranda, a Latin American exile with whom he was often to be seen 'descanting about art'. Miranda – whom Dr James Barry was later to acknowledge as her mentor – made a striking contrast to the bohemian little artist: a Venezuelan by birth, he had dedicated his life to the cause of revolution in whatever corner of the globe it appeared. As a soldier and a scholar he had travelled widely and had been the lover of Catherine the Great and Madame de Staël – in fact it was said of him that he 'fascinated women from Constantinople to Charleston'. Cultured, worldly, and a Catholic, like Barry he shared many interests with his friend – not least an appreciation of women's company. It seems very possible that the two radical, free-thinking men shared the favours of at least one courtesan: indeed, when the chance of liberating his native land recalled Miranda to South America in 1805, he left his mistress under the artist's protection.

Given the influence that Miranda undoubtedly exerted over Dr James Barry during the early years of her life, one cannot ignore the possibility that he may – like her 'uncle' – have been her real father. So little concrete evidence survives that no reasonable candidate can be discounted. But it seems far more likely that the little girl who was to become Dr James Barry was in fact the artist's niece, the younger of two daughters of Mary Ann Bulkley, *née* Barry. In the spring of 1805 Mrs Bulkley travelled from Cork to London to beg for help for herself and her girls, Margaret, who was nearly 15, and a much younger child, unknown and unnamed. . . . She had been pleading for her brother's help throughout the previous year since she was destitute, 'thrown out of house and home' shortly after her husband's bankruptcy. What caused the rift is unknown, but plainly Mary Anne felt sufficiently desperate to appeal to a brother she had not seen for thirty years.

The artist's response was discouraging; when his eldest niece Margaret came to see him she received scant courtesy. Mary Anne wrote reproachfully from lodgings,

What did you give my child? Did you ask her to dinner? Did you act as an uncle or a Christian to a poor unprotected, unprovided for girl who had not been brought up to think of labour and, alas, whose education is not finished to put herself in a way to get decent bread for herself, and whose share has been given to a brother?

In fact the artist was in no position to help his relatives. Always hopelessly maladroit where money matters were concerned, he was by now almost entirely without means; his scathing attacks on the staff of the Royal Academy where he had held a post as Professor of Painting had finally led to his dismissal and he was reduced to making etchings of his own work in the hope of selling them. He was now living in a wretched, tumbledown house with broken windows, without 'a servant or a decent bed'.

But if her brother proved unable to help, at least Mary Anne found his friends more accommodating. In particular General Miranda quickly took an interest in the Bulkley family. Perhaps this vigorous man in his early fifties was attracted by the shrewd, determined Irish woman; in any case it was natural that he should be drawn to her little daughter who already showed a precocious love of books and an instinct for learning. He consented to entertain the family in his tasteful rooms in Bloomsbury and, more surprisingly, to allow the youngest to finger his precious volumes. It was said of Miranda that he had the most remarkable collection of books in London – among them 'a list of tomes to form a tolerably complete medical library for a private gentleman who is not of the profession'.

But his influence on the little girl did not stop there: when guests came to call she was allowed to peep at the assembled company from behind the curtains.

And what a brilliant company it was – statesmen and scholars, grand ladies and diplomats came to dine off French china and silver dishes. Fine wines were served to the company but General Miranda himself usually drank sweetened water, his favourite beverage. His gatherings were above all intellectual occasions: as in the great days of the blue-stockings, when guests were invited to 'come in their day clothes' and cards were prohibited, brilliant conversation flourished. A Danish poet declared that 'a visitor might indeed believe himself in the Athens of Pericles'.

After Miranda's departure to America in September 1805, a new and even more idiosyncratic protector began to interest himself in the family. Lord Buchan had for years been a friend and patron of James Barry; an incurable snob who liked to address the king as 'my dear cousin' he nevertheless had a genuine – if somewhat undisciplined – passion for art. He was regarded by his friends as something of an eccentric – in addition to his devoted (if sometimes unwelcome) support of artistic talent he was an ardent feminist. He named ladies as his literary executors and in 1791, the year before Mary Wollstonecraft published her well-known *Vindication Of The Rights Of Women*, had written an impassioned plea for female education:

> Let us consider for a few minutes . . . the consequences that have arisen from the barbarous education of women in all ages as playthings or housekeepers for gentlemen of fortune . . . and we shall be able to see at a glance that the whole female code of education must be changed . . . before it can be proved that women in the present state of civilised society should have in almost every respect as truly learned institutions as men . . . The men of Europe have crushed the heads of women in their infancy and then laugh at them because their brains are not so well ordered as they desire.

Throughout 1805 Buchan wrote endless letters in his effort to obtain an annuity for Barry; he even asked the artist's permission to set up a small sub-committee within the Royal Society of Arts to procure him 'a proper residence' where he could fulfil his genius 'without interruption and insult'. But he was to be disappointed. In February of the following year, while dining at a favourite Soho haunt, James Barry was seized with pains in his chest; he died a few days later. The funeral, in St Paul's Cathedral, was in striking contrast to the poverty in which he had lived: seventeen coaches attended the hearse-and-four as it drove from Adam Street to the Cathedral.

The pageantry of his funeral can have been of little comfort to his relatives, but Buchan was determined that they should not suffer. In June the same year the *Gentleman's Magazine* reported that he was collecting James Barry's manuscript works and drawings: 'with an intention to publish them for the advantage of some indigent relatives of the departed artist'. Miranda, now back in England after an unsuccessful attempt to invade Venezuela, was helping him with the project, and Dr Fryer, a prominent physician, was to write the text.

But the three friends' collaboration had another and more important purpose. They had decided that Mary Anne Bulkley's younger daughter, whose outstanding intellectual abilities were by now obvious, should have an education worthy of her. The problem was how to provide it: by virtue of her sex the little girl was barred from every university in the country. However brilliant she was, without qualifications her talents would never find their proper fulfilment: at best she could look forward to the frustrations of life as a governess. Then there was the financial aspect. As a woman her comfort and security would depend on making a wealthy marriage, with all the restrictions on her development that would imply. And her fortune, such as it was, had long ago been made over to her brother in Ireland, the family 'favourite'.

We can never know at what point the obvious, but incredible solution suggested itself. But by 1809 little Miss Bulkley had exchanged her skirts for breeches and, accompanied by her mother, was starting the long coach journey northwards to enrol as a medical student at Edinburgh University. Edinburgh had been chosen because Buchan held considerable influence there; the medical faculty because it offered the most advanced scientific education available. The danger of discovery would be ever present, but her three friends stood ready to help at every turn. With her new name, James Barry was assuming more than a professional identity; she was beginning a career that would come to dominate her entire life.

2

On Record

When James Barry, 'literary and medical student', signed the Matriculation Roll of Edinburgh University in December 1809 she was a phenomenon. A ten-year-old girl, dressed in boys' clothes, entering a university which even forty-six years later refused to allow Sophia Jex-Blake to study in medical classes with men.

The idea of a ten-year-old entering university was not quite as unbelievable as it sounds today. To matriculate in those days merely required a payment of two shillings and sixpence for a ticket to the university library; the classes themselves resembled school. Indeed, in the eighteenth century it was not uncommon for boys of twelve to become students at Edinburgh. Two well-known examples are Sir Walter Scott and David Hume. But while students of the Humanities often attended without the slightest intention of taking a degree, it was clear from the beginning that little James Barry intended to take her M.D. As a medical student she had to write her thesis and 'defend' it orally in Latin.

The course took three years and she studied ferociously. She settled in with Mrs Bulkley in lodgings at Number 6, Lothian Street, Edinburgh, in one of the grey granite streets near the Medical School. In her first year she took not only the requisite courses in the curriculum – chemistry, botany, anatomy, medical jurisprudence, Greek, natural and moral philosophy – but also two optional subjects. She attended the crowded classes in midwifery held by Dr Hamilton, a gruff Scot and leading obstetrician who supported the town's lying-in hospital at his own expense and refused to deliver the babies of great ladies in the country. 'Let them come to me,' he would growl. Dissection, her other extra subject, she studied as a private pupil with Mr Fyfe, one of the last Edinburgh physicians to sport a pigtail and a typical eccentric of the time. Mr Fyfe, a 'horrid' lecturer, but a good practical anatomist, personally supervised all the dissections and after classes he liked to chat to the students around the fireside.

At the beginning of the nineteenth century, Edinburgh was an exciting city – 'the Athens of the North' – with its new broad streets and its cosmopolitan population. The Medical School already had a fine reputation and Barry's class roll shows that her fellow students came from as far afield as the West Indies, America and India.

Among her classmates James Barry was withdrawn. She was slight and small (barely five foot tall) and 'apparently of delicate constitution . . . vain and could be frivolous, yet was prompt to resent an offence'.

Barry's life with Mrs Bulkley was sheltered and secretive. Obviously she could not attend those student societies where 'lords, lawyers and lairds' met to down a gill of brandy at four when dinner was on the table, and stayed up carousing until the small hours. Sedate Sunday afternoons with Dr Duncan, her lecturer in medical jurisprudence, who invited twenty or thirty students every week for a 'dull enough tea and talk' party, were more suitable for her entertainment. And a note of gaiety is, understandably, missing from her student days. Reading was, perhaps, the only pastime allowed her, and one of her books, a novel entitled *The Miseries of Human Life or the Groans of Timothy Testly and Samuel Sensitive*, by James Beresford, published in Edinburgh in 1807, hints at her taste in light reading.

That James Barry kept her classmates at a distance is hardly surprising. However, she did make friends with one student, a lad named Jobson. He recalled, years later, what a figure of fun she cut, wrapped up in her long 'surtout', in contrast to the other students who sported shooting coats.

To Jobson's astonishment he found that James Barry was afraid to venture alone through the rougher parts of town. Although Jobson too was small in stature, he was a keen sportsman and he decided to teach Barry the rudiments of boxing. But he discovered to his disappointment that 'James Barry would never strike out but always kept his arms over his chest'. In spite of this, Jobson did not suspect Barry's sex.

For her part she evidently trusted Jobson enough to invite him to her lodgings. There he was introduced to her 'mother', Mrs Bulkley. This was surprising, since Barry always referred to Mrs Bulkley as her 'aunt'. In fact, in one of the most revealing letters she ever wrote, she made a point of underlining the relationship. The letter was addressed to General Miranda and dated January 1810, a few weeks after she joined the university.

In a letter I had the honour of receiving from my inestimable friend Dr Fryer, he says that in consequence of your kind enquiries about my pursuits etc. he did not conceal from so particular a friend of my late uncle's any circumstance relative to my successore [? fortunes]; I am truly grateful for the communication and I think I may congratulate myself on being thought of by so very eminent a man.

The last day of the year I dined at the Earl Buchan's who said General Miranda was known to him not only by fame but that he had been introduced to him on his arrival in this country. I could not help telling his Lordship what a Treasure you possess in London and how often you permitted me (Barry's nephew) to partake it, it is needless to say I mean your very extensive and elegant Library – of my part I am studying and attending the Greek, Natural Philosophy, Chemistry, and Anatomy Classes and am honoured by the notice of the above mentioned earl and of Dr Munro the celebrated professor of Anatomy. The Doctor speaks of you whom he knows by Fame and of Dr Fryer whose correspondence with Lord B – his particular friend he has read with Enthusiasm – Excuse my troubling you with this letter, but I could not deny myself the pleasure of wishing you very many happy returns of the New Year in which Mrs Bulkley (my aunt) joins with me.

I must beg the favour, when you see Dr Fryer, to tell him that Lord Buchan desires me to say that we drank his health at his house in George Street this day week.

As Lord B – nor anyone else here knows anything about Mrs Bulkley's Daughter, I trust, my dear General, that neither you nor the Doctor will mention in any of your correspondence anything of my Cousin's friendship and Ca for me.

A remarkable letter for a little girl, albeit an extraordinarily gifted little girl, to write, granted the stilted and grandiloquent style of educated children in those days. Throughout that letter, she seems to have been reminding General Miranda of her role. 'You permitted me (Barry's nephew) . . . Mrs Bulkley (my aunt).' And then the extraordinary postscript.

It is difficult to understand this letter and General Miranda's interest in the young medical student unless her future was of considerable importance to him. Miranda valued his books above all his possessions. He kept his library under lock and key, and lit fires in the room in July to keep it at a constant temperature; permission to handle the books was a sign of special favour.

From Barry's letter one can deduce that her relationship with Miranda was elaborately disguised. She writes of Lord Buchan as if he was a stranger to him and yet the two had collaborated to ensure the success of Dr Fryer's life of James Barry, R.A. The two men were united in their concern for the relatives of the artist. Perhaps Barry herself was not aware of the plotting that took place among her uncle's friends.

All one can say for certain is that her life was cloaked in secrecy. Only study seems to have offered a means of escape. Until the summer of 1810, Mrs Bulkley stayed with her (which of course set her apart from other students). Then her friend and patron, Lord Buchan, took charge. In July 1810 he wrote to Dr Robert Anderson, Scottish scholar and editor, whose home was a centre of Scottish literary life, to thank him for agreeing to take Barry as a lodger.

I cannot but greatly approve in the expression of your kindness to poor Barry and your willingness to take him under your care as a Boarder when Mrs Bulkley leaves Scotland.

Considering the friendship which subsisted between Barry's uncle and myself and other circumstances I have taken the liberty of recommending him more particularly to your attention as you will see by the two Billets which I send enclosed to your care . . .

Maddeningly, the two billets with the details of the 'other circumstances' are missing from the archives of the Scottish National Library.

Perhaps it was fortunate that Barry was too busy for introspection. By 1811 she had added practice of physic, theory of medicine and literary classes to her already crowded syllabus. She had also decided to attend a course in Military Surgery. At that stage it was not her intention to join the British Army although the Napoleonic Wars were at their height. Barry meant to go 'by invitation of General Miranda' to Caracas and she was working hard to prepare herself. In 1811 she became a perpetual student at the Royal Infirmary, Dispensary and Lying-In Hospital in Edinburgh. One gains some idea of how hectic life was from a letter written home almost forty years earlier by a student at the same hospital.

Rose at 7, read till 9, breakfasted at 9, attended lectures, transcribed notes, from 12 to 1 walked wards, from 1 to 3 in anatomical department. Dined in lodgings 3–5. Attended midwifery lecture 6–7. Attended anatomical demonstrations. Supped at 9 p.m. and worked till midnight.

During the summer holidays, Lord Buchan, indefatigable on Barry's behalf, invited her to stay at his home in Dryburgh Abbey, set in pleasant wooded country near the Tweed. She spent most of her five-week visit working in the Earl's extensive library. Since she was working during her vacation, one gains the impression that she was under great pressure to finish her studies and gain her degree. When she returned to Edinburgh she took with her another letter from Buchan addressed to Dr Anderson stating that 'James Barry . . . has employed himself in my library very busily in useful reading of Books connected with his professional views'. (Dr Anderson, of course, knew perfectly well by then who James Barry was.) But Buchan seemed unable to resist the melodrama in the affair: 'He is a well disposed young man and worthy of your notice and advice in his studies', he continued, and went on to ask Dr Anderson and his son-in-law Dr Irving to 'look into the Latinity of his thesis'. Barry, noted Buchan, was 'much younger than is usual to take a degree in Medicine and surgery yet from what I have observed likely to entitle himself to them by his attainments'.

At the age of twelve she completed her thesis 'De Merocele' on hernia of the groin. The Senate refused to admit her to the degree examination because of her extreme youth, but again Lord Buchan intervened and pointed out that there were no regulations governing the minimum age of degree candidates.

The Senate relented and she passed brilliantly. On the frontispiece of her thesis she quoted from Menander in the Greek: 'Do not consider my youth, but consider whether I show a man's wisdom': it is a plea that sounds heartfelt from a lonely secretive girl. Her dedication to *Francisco Miranda* was in the florid Latin style that was customary; she extolled his praises and offered thanks for his 'paternal care'. She also made a more restrained dedication to her patron, *David Steuart Erskine*, Earl of Buchan. Significantly, she signed her name in her school books 'James Miranda Steuart Barry'.

By qualifying as a doctor James Barry had proved to herself and to the remarkable circle which protected her that, given the opportunity, a woman could become the intellectual equal of a man. So far she had stood up to the strain remarkably well. But student days had shown that to maintain her disguise she had to pay the price of terrible isolation. On the positive side Barry displayed a high seriousness towards the professional responsibilities she had earned at such a cost. From now on she would become most sure of her own role when working as a doctor; her skill and compassion were to win respect wherever she went.

By October 1812 Barry had moved to London. As a Pupil Dresser at St Thomas's Hospital and an apprentice to Sir Astley Cooper, a leading London surgeon, she held a privileged position. Sir Astley, who later operated on George IV, was regarded as the finest teacher in the profession. His classes attracted crowds. When he stepped down from his carriage at Guy's Hospital hundreds of students jostled on the steps to see the maestro appear in his blue coat and yellow buckskin breeches, his massive well-proportioned legs hosed in silk stockings. But for all his grand appearance Sir Astley preferred to live in Broad Street, near the large warehouse where he kept his 'subjects', bodies stolen from the poorer graveyards nearby. The Professor of Anatomy at Guy's was required to lecture and dissect the bodies of executed criminals, but the supply was not always adequate, and Sir Astley was quite ready to supplement it from other sources. Although the authorities knew of his stealthy activities, Sir Astley kept his windows blacked over to avoid offending the neighbours.

Barry must have felt drawn to this outstanding doctor. Sir Astley was a man of wide interests and such radical views that as a young man he had crossed to France as a sympathizer with the Revolution at the same time that General Miranda was actually fighting there. However, on his appointment to the staff of Guy's Hospital in 1800, he had been obliged to temper his politics.

Through his work, Sir Astley raised the prestige of his profession. He was a brilliant innovator as well as a skilful surgeon. In 1816 he performed the first ligation of the aorta for aneurysm. Most important of all from Dr Barry's point of view, Sir Astley approached medicine as scientifically as the age would allow.

'In disease', he lectured, 'medical men guess; if they cannot ascertain a disease they call it nervous.' Sir Astley impressed upon his students the importance of careful observation: 'Nothing is known in our profession by guess. There is no short road to knowledge. The way to learn your profession is to look for yourself.'

Sir Astley was a country man, a practical man and when he described disease he would show his students examples of afflicted patients. He illustrated the theory of physiology, pathology and surgery with drawings, paintings, dissections and operations. Many of his students became outstanding medical men. He was a compassionate practitioner and an inspiring teacher, always ready with advice: 'A surgeon', he would remind his pupils in his broad Norfolk accent, 'should have an eagle's eye, a lady's hand and a lion's heart.' He might almost have been describing Barry.

Pupil Dressers at the time paid a fee of £50 a year for their apprenticeship. The fee entitled them not only to witness the dissection of all morbid bodies in the dead house, but also to watch their teacher operating at top speed on his groaning, semiconscious patients. Although some students fainted at the sight and the stench of dead bodies, Barry must have fought down her nausea to study intently. She retained a quick sympathy for suffering throughout her career yet she always endured the screams, the blood, and the dirt of the hospitals.

For six months, until the spring of 1813, Barry walked the wards. By then she must have heard the news of General Miranda's imprisonment in a Puerto Rican gaol, his dream of liberating Venezuela broken. For her it meant the end of a dream too. She could not escape to the anonymity of South America. She could not join Miranda. She had to find another means of practising medicine where she would be fairly safe from discovery. On the Continent the Napoleonic Wars were raging. The Army, inefficient and corrupt in peacetime, was gaining glory from Wellington's victories and news of the campaign was spread through town and village by laurel-wreathed coaches. But with the victories came the inevitable toll of wounded: the Army needed doctors.

Largely as the result of the work of Dr James McGrigor, Wellington's Principal Medical Officer, the profession had won a new status. Before Barry's time the old barber-surgeons, mere servants of the Colonels, had been replaced by educated men. In 1811, the year before she passed her final examination, the Horse Guards gave orders that physicians were to be chosen only from Regimental and Staff Surgeons with an M.D. from a British university. They were rare enough.

In the summer of 1813, Barry and her student friend Dr Jobson went to Fort Pitt, Chatham, the army depot. They had decided to enlist together.

Perhaps Barry had been persuaded by her influential friends that to enter the Army on the hospital staff would provide her with the best chance of protection and promotion. The Army Medical Department at that time was divided into a regimental section which travelled with the troops in the field and a staff section where the doctors enjoyed permanent quarters and a degree of privacy. Also she would spend most of her life abroad, away from London and the danger of discovery.

Physical examinations in those days were perfunctory, involving perhaps opening one waistcoat button. Distaste for allowing a physician to examine the patient without clothes was so extreme that Duchesses relayed their symptoms via ladies' maids – sometimes with disastrous results. Soon after Victoria came to the throne, Lady Flora Hastings, a Lady-in-Waiting at the Court, was thought to be in an 'interesting condition'. In fact she had an enlarged liver but rather than permit the Queen's physician Sir James Clark to examine her 'with her stays removed' she endured weeks of malicious Court gossip. Only when the Queen herself intervened did Lady Flora consent to a full examination. Whether or not influential friends intervened to prevent Dr Barry from having to submit to a 'medical' is not clear. But when she sat for her army exam, doctors of her calibre with both an Edinburgh degree and experience as Pupil Dresser to a leading London surgeon were badly needed and this in itself may have exempted her. 'I entered the Army under the age of fourteen,' she wrote with obvious pride in numerous official documents. On the 5th of July Dr James Barry was gazetted Hospital Assistant – the most junior commissioned officer in the Medical Department of the Army.

She went straight to the Hospital of the Plymouth garrison and escaped the rough and tumble of mess life that she would have had to endure as a regimental surgeon. She was still under fourteen. A slight girl in scarlet tunic and tight breeches, she had high cheeks, reddish hair, large rather haunted blue eyes and a prominent nose. Her mouth already held a scornful twist.

With her large sword and spurs, and cocked hat with tassels and feathers, she must have presented an extraordinary figure to the medical officer in charge. Dr Skey protested at the youthful appearance of the new recruit but received word that 'it was not wise to agitate the question'.

Lord Buchan, always ready to champion her, wrote to Dr Anderson from Dryburgh Abbey in November that he had recommended Barry to Dr Skey. He enclosed a 'letter relating to poor James Barry'. After a good deal of trouble deciphering Skey's handwriting Lord Buchan had discovered that Barry had 'found favour with his principal whom I intend to thank for his attentions and request the continuance of them . . .'

A curious silence, considering all the public attention she was soon to arouse, surrounds Barry's next two years in the Army. Only a faint pencilled entry in an early Register of Medical Officers records her station as Stoke. Stoke Park belonged to the Duchess of Beaufort, mother of Lord Charles Somerset, second son of the Duke of Beaufort. Lord Charles was Commander-in-Chief and Governor of the Cape of Good Hope; Lord Fitzroy Somerset, his younger brother (later Lord

Raglan) held great influence in the Army. Was it pure coincidence that Dr James Barry, gazetted as Assistant Surgeon to the Forces, was posted to the Cape in 1816, where Lord Charles was in command? For Lord Charles Somerset too had family ties that reached back to the world of the blue-stocking and the literati where the Barry plot had been planned. Sixty years earlier his maternal grandmother, the Hon. Mrs Boscawen, had been equally at home in the company of the writers and artists of the day, with their frank speech and casual dress, as in the powdered and painted world she had been born to.

By all accounts she was a remarkable woman: 'her manners are the most agreeable and her conversation the best of any lady with whom I have had the happiness to be acquainted', wrote Boswell in his life of Dr Johnson. David Garrick and Edmund Burke also numbered among her intimates: as a young politician Burke counted on her friendship so closely that he hoped to gain preferment with Pitt through mentioning her name. Strangely enough, Burke also had a remarkably close connection with the Barry family, both with the artist and his father, a Sea Captain who plied the Bristol to Cork route. Through him, Mrs Boscawen and John Barry almost certainly met. John Barry fathered a daughter long after his wife had passed childbearing age. In the parish records the name of the mother is missing: could it have been Mrs Boscawen? If Juliana Barry (later Mary Anne Bulkley) was indeed Mrs Boscawen's daughter that would explain the Beaufort connection – and hence Barry's posting to the Cape.

Even if Dr James Barry was not Mrs Boscawen's granddaughter – and it can never be proved – she could rely on more than a dynastic loyalty from the Beauforts. She was a child of the circle and when she went out to the Cape she was assured of a special welcome.

3

Quite a Prodigy

'I suffered greatly from sea voyages', wrote Barry at the close of her career. On her first journey to the Cape she was forced to spend almost three months aboard a sailing ship, cramped and uncomfortable, her privacy under threat.

At sea she disliked the monotonous diet of boiled mutton or boiled pork. She missed fresh milk, fresh fruit and fresh vegetables, all foods highly prized by her. When hurricane-force winds buffeted the ship, she fell prey to seasickness. It must have been a great relief to sight land at last. She stepped ashore in August 1816, jaunty and confident despite the weeks of discomfort. She soon made her appearance in the streets of Cape Town, kitted out in full dress uniform scarlet tunic, cocked hat with feathers and a sword almost bigger than herself. She wore soles three inches thick in her boots and high heels to boost her tiny figure; her shoulders, so the natives swore, were padded with cotton wool.

Trotting down the straight, tree-lined streets of the Cape on her pony, with a black servant carrying a sunshade at her side and a poodle yapping at her heels, she seemed almost to court discovery. With her sword and spurs gleaming, her tiny figure erect and proud, she evidently enjoyed the display and the comment her appearance provoked. Dressing up in full army regalia perhaps allowed Barry to revel in the deception. So many stories about James Barry vary so wildly, yet impressions of her appearance generally agree. She must have made an extraordinary little figure. One shrewd observer noticed that she walked with her elbows tucked in instead of out.

The first breath of suspicion about her sex came, soon after she arrived, from a naval man. Captain William Henry Dillon of H.M.S. *Horatio* had anchored in Simon's Bay, Cape Town, on his way home from China. He soon needed medical treatment. 'The ship had not been long at anchor when I was attacked by a violent inflammation in both eyes, the result of a cold caught in the late gales', wrote the Captain. Despite the attentions of the ship's surgeon – he even opened the Captain's right temple – the inflammation and the pain persisted.

Captain Dillon wrote,

As I suffered so much I applied to the family physician of the Governor, Lord Charles Somerset. This gentleman was in the Army and considered extremely clever. Many surmises were in circulation relating to him; from the awkwardness of his gait and the shape of his person it was the prevailing opinion that he was a female.

Barely a month in the Cape and gossip already rife. What is worth noting is that this account was published during Barry's lifetime, in 1856, before suspicions were openly voiced.

The Captain also noted that Dr Barry 'was extremely assiduous but did not approve the remedies resorted to, plainly telling me a milder treatment would have sufficed. Having written down his instructions and explained fully the system I was to follow, he took his leave and demanded only his travelling expenses to the ship and back.'

That a seventeen-year-old girl had the confidence and the skill that Barry displayed is difficult to grasp. With a brilliant brain, a splendid uniform and her medical knowledge, she could hold her ground with anyone.

More than a year before she was officially appointed Physician to the Governor, Barry, in effect, held that office. From the moment she arrived, she attended the Governor and his family personally. She was a constant companion to the ruddy, handsome widower and his teenage daughters. Her intimacy with the Somerset family gained her immediate acceptance into the snobbish circle surrounding the Governor – but it also aroused some envy. The Governor ruled the Colony despotically. His favourites prospered and as a result jealousy and gossip dogged their footsteps.

Of the 15 000 settlers in Cape Town in those years, the modish officers of the garrison led society, with the senior civil functionaries, the Dutch lawyers and the rich farmers and slave-hirers close behind. In descending order in the hierarchy of that time came the Indians, with the Malays, and then the Hottentots and blacks. Although it was illegal to land slaves in a British port after 1807, the practice continued. Slaves imported in this manner were termed 'prize Negroes' and apprenticed to tradesmen and officials.

From the outset, one of Barry's blind spots as far as Cape society was concerned was her apparent disregard of the Colony's racial divisions. She would actually ask her black patients direct questions and very much upset the prison authorities in the Randbosch some years later by questioning the black prisoners about their diet and hygiene in gaol. (The white settlers had, in any case, not proved very co-operative. 'Why', they asked, 'do you ask blacks questions, while Christians are present to answer?')

The early years were on the whole happy, active and full of interest. She lived in lodgings owned by a widow in one of the white, flat-roofed houses on the Herrengracht, the most prominent street in Cape Town. A few doors along, at Society House, the colonists read three- or four-month-old newspapers from home, drank coffee, played billiards or simply watched the world go by.

Every one seems to remember that Barry bought buns for Psyche, her poodle, from Mrs Saunders' confectionery shop in the Herrengracht. She always lived in a certain style, with a black or Malay servant, and from the beginning she gave strict orders that no one was to enter her bedroom. Psyche, her inseparable companion, slept on her bed – for company or to warn her mistress of danger . . .

And danger of discovery seems to have been very close in those first months at the Cape. In January 1817 she was called on professionally to visit a distinguished stranger, a prisoner in apartments in the old Dutch Castle. She went along with a Sea Captain from St Helena where Napoleon was exiled.

When he saw Barry, the distinguished prisoner was confused. 'I mistook the Captain's medical friend for his son or nephew. The grave doctor who was presented to me was a boy of 18, *with the form, the manners and the voice of a woman* . . .'

Count de Las Casas, the writer, was a shrewd and worldly observer, the father of a seventeen-year-old boy himself, a loyal supporter of Napoleon who had followed the Emperor into exile on St Helena.

The Count had spent his time in exile as Napoleon's amanuensis, taking down the great man's ideas and recollections and using his own son, Emmanuel, to write up the notes. But father and son were intercepted trying to smuggle out secret messages to Napoleon's supporters in England, written in a minute hand on the silk lining of a waistcoat. As a result they were both shipped off to the Cape in January 1817 under close arrest.

Dr Barry was asked to examine Emmanuel de Las Casas, the Count's son. She found him suffering from nothing more serious than lack of exercise and fresh air, and prescribed baths and regular physical exertion. The prisoners were housed in the dungeon of the Castle in Cape Town and water could not be procured. Nevertheless in Barry the pair found a friend and Count de Las Casas noted in his journal that she was regarded as 'an absolute phenomenon. I was informed that he had obtained his diploma at the age of thirteen after the most rigid examination; that he had performed extraordinary cures at the Cape and had saved the life of one of the Governor's daughters after she had been given up, which rendered him a sort of favourite in the family.'

Lord Charles Somerset, the Governor, publicly expressed his confidence in the very young, odd-looking little doctor. Writing to Earl Bathurst, Secretary of State for the Colonies, to assure him that he was taking good care of the prisoners, he said: 'I furnish him [Las Casas] with the best medical attention. Dr Barry (who attends my own family) has constantly prescribed for him.' (Plainly, the fascination and awe still generally felt for Napoleon left the British Government in some doubt as to whether to treat the Emperor and his supporters as dangerous prisoners or diplomatic visitors.)

Barry proved a valuable advocate for Las Casas. Because the Count was worried about his son he wrote to the Governor begging permission to allow the boy to go to Europe. The request touched Lord Charles's strong sense of family and he consented, but Emmanuel refused to leave his father.

The Count then asked Dr Barry to exert her professional influence.

> But instead of listening to me [Barry] hastened to Emmanuel's chamber and embracing him, expressed his approval of his conduct, observing that he should not have respected him had he done otherwise. Conducting [Emmanuel] to the window he introduced the boy to the two ladies whom he had left in their carriage. The Misses Somerset brought Barry as far as the courtyard, curious to see the prisoner.

Barry was more aware of the loneliness of life without a family than most people of her age. Emmanuel, only a year her junior, would have brought her own situation to mind.

Throughout her life Barry always identified herself with people in prison. The people she cared about, the people who had influenced her – the artist Barry, General Miranda (who had died in a Spanish prison in 1816), even the eccentric Earl of Buchan – all held lofty, sometimes grandiose ideas about freedom and liberty. Was she herself not a prisoner of an impossible situation, forced to masquerade in order to fulfil her vocation, as a doctor?

In Barry, Count de Las Casas recognized an ally. She was the only stranger he ever saw. He found her company 'very agreeable' and noted that she 'could guess the seat of my disorder and regretted that it was out of his power to prescribe any remedy for me, a prisoner in a dungeon'.

Barry, in fact, did find a temporary solution for Las Casas. Lord Charles was embarking on a tour of the eastern frontier of the Colony at the end of January 1817, and Barry persuaded the Governor to house the Count and Emmanuel in one of his country houses while he was away. Newlands was a splendid mansion 'two leagues from Cape Town', with large, lofty rooms and elegant gardens – a paradise after the Castle.

Since gossip already existed about the friendship between Assistant Staff Surgeon Barry and the lordly Governor, no one was surprised to learn that Lord Charles included the diminutive doctor in his suite on tour, as well as the Deputy Colonial Secretary, Colonel Bird, and Captain Thomas Sheridan, the Colonial Treasurer (who owed his position to his playwright father's friendship with the Prince Regent).

The tour lasted three months and they travelled in the grandest manner. Lord Charles was used to extravagant living and even in the bush was not prepared to live rough. Nevertheless, they had to jolt over 500 miles of rough cart-tracks, stifling in the dust and the heat in the huge, creaking ox-drawn wagons. But the sights they saw compensated for the discomfort. They passed through magnificent country, glimpsing elephants, the occasional rhinoceros and large grey vultures. At night jackals and wolves howled and the Hottentots sang and played on crude violins by the camp fire. One night, a small Hottentot boy in charge of a team of oxen fell asleep and was snatched up by a lion on the prowl. The boy's screams roused the camp; the lion dropped his prey and slunk into the bush. Barry examined the boy to make sure he was suffering from nothing more serious than shock and, to the surprise of the natives, attended to him with the same care she would have shown to a white man.

On the coast they stopped at the very British village of Knysna. Its squire, George Rex, rode to hounds in pink coat with his own pack and lived in a fine manor house, Melkhout Kraal, flanked by formal tree-lined avenues. The thatched, whitewashed farms outside the village overlooked an exotic lagoon where flamingos flocked. Mr Rex owned 100 slaves and 25 000 acres and he entertained his guests lavishly with fishing and shooting parties and dinners at the great mansion. He was rumoured to be the son of George III and the Quaker Hannah Lightfoot and he personally approved all the original settlers at Knysna. The Royal Navy even had a station there. It was rare for the family to have a visitor as cultivated as Barry and she spent much of her visit reading to the young Rexes (of whom there were eight at that time). At Featherbed Bay close by lay the ship of Sir Jahleel Brenton, the Naval Commissioner at Simonstown, and one night the whole party were invited to dine on board. Sir Jahleel was a man of great piety, fiercely opposed to slavery, and he and Barry discovered an affinity. This casual acquaintance struck up in an African village was to prove a valuable support to her in the years to come.

Despite the discomfort, the trek must have been a marvellous experience. As the party approached the frontier, passing through lush, green park-like country, local magistrates joined

Lord Charles's party – the Landrost of Uitenhage, with a contingent of 100 dragoons, complete with artillery and two field pieces, and the Landrost of Graaf Reinet escorted by a home guard of 350 burghers. This show of military strength designed to impress the natives and discourage them from molesting the settlers almost defeated its purpose. So alarmed were the tribesmen, armed only with assegais, at the sight of the howitzer guns and the grand marquee surrounded on all sides by redcoated troops, that some fled to the hills. They were finally persuaded to return when a Government official and a British officer went to meet Gaika, the Kaffir chief, and his uncle Ndhlambie, who came accompanied by a guard of about 300 warriors.

The natives met the white man in the shape of the magnificently attired Governor, Colonel Bird, Captain Sheridan – and the pocket-sized Dr James Barry.

Amid much courtly ceremony, a system of protection for the colonists' cattle was worked out and a plan was agreed for establishing a series of military posts to police the frontier. Exchange and barter were also encouraged, and, as a gesture of goodwill, Lord Charles presented Gaika with a fine grey horse and a sack of shoes, handkerchiefs, buttons, knives, beads, looking glasses and tinder boxes. At the end of April, the party came home exhausted, to rest for a few days at Newlands, Lord Charles's country seat.

It is hard to estimate Barry's influence on the Governor in her first years at the Cape but it must have been considerable. The need for a colony for the lepers who wandered about in rags, starving, shunned and feared, was voiced in 1815 before her arrival. In 1817, after she had been at the Cape less than a year, the colony at Hemel and Aarde (Heaven and Earth) in the Caledon District, was founded.

The contrasts of life at the Cape in those days were staggering. Infanticide was common and barely caused comment; black babies were frequently found dead on the beach. Life was cheap. The farmers worked or flogged their slaves to exhaustion. The Hottentots, Malays and Negroes lived in squalor and misery; those who were sick were sent to prison.

Conditions in the mother country were not much better, but at least a parliament, which was soon to become more representative, had been established. At the Cape, governed by Roman

Dutch Law, the Governor was still a despot. Most of the English colonists and the Dutch burghers lived in Cape Town in fine old houses with fragrant gardens. They seemed able to ignore misery and cruelty to the natives as easily as they ignored the filth and stench from the canals as they drove past in their smart curricles or phaetons.

James Barry was well aware that, on at least three counts, she could never be one of them. She was a woman masquerading as a man – an unheard of impropriety; she was a Roman Catholic who felt bound to conceal her faith to conform with army practice; and she had been born out of wedlock. Small wonder that she showed compassion and particular sympathy towards those whom society shunned.

The frustrations and indignations of her own life must have found some release in helping the slaves. She actually freed one boy, Hermes, who was just about to be sent to prison for a petty theft, committed while he was the property of a typically tyrannical Dutch householder. Barry paid the family the ransom for Hermes and placed the Hottentot boy safely in Sir Jahleel Brenton's household where he became a family favourite.

Yet she enjoyed the life in the Colony. She was young. She was popular. She was talented. Visits to the theatre, excursions to the races and days out hunting with the Somerset family formed part of her round: Lord Charles was a gentleman jockey and passionately fond of the horses. Off duty, Barry was in demand at parties and balls, a witty conversationalist dressed immaculately in a 'coat of the latest pea-green Hayne', a satin waistcoat and a pair of tight-fitting 'inexpressibles' (knee breeches). She danced well, and always took care to be seen with the prettiest girls in the room. In fact she deliberately made herself a reputation as a 'lady-killer'.

One might have thought that, in her position, Barry would have tried to efface herself. Quite the contrary. She seems to have had a gift for attracting attention, and perhaps to have enjoyed the sensation. One Lois Chance, writing to a Cape paper in the 1880s, recalled talks with her grandmother (Barry's patient) in a vivid pen-picture. At a dance on board the flagship of a squadron her grandmother met Dr Barry, a 'perfect dancer who won his way to many a heart with impeccable bedroom manners. In fact he was a flirt – I expect this was one of the many affectations designed to avert suspicion. He had a winning way with women . . . and his beautiful small white hands were the envy of many a lady of that date.'

Barry was staying with the Governor's party at Alphen overnight (on the outskirts of the Cape). 'The next day my grandmother was overcome: excitement had brought on an attack of nerves . . . Barry promptly sent her to bed, much to her chagrin. The following morning, very early, Dr Barry came to her room, booted and spurred, ready for the hunt.' His touch was gentle and his voice in a sick room was kind and low. As he left the room, my grandmother remarked to her body-servant, 'It might have been a woman touching my head: the doctor's hands are so light.'

Of all the extravaganza written about Barry after her death, that simple account seems to ring true. But the young doctor, a brilliant diagnostician, firm and kind in the sickroom (although scathing and quick-tempered with malingerers or slapdash colleagues) was a splendid sportsman. She was in the fore at a hunt, a superb marksman and an accomplished four-in-hand whip. She could often be seen driving her carriage with four high-spirited greys through broad streets of the town.

She was fond of a racy story and a glass of wine and her gaiety quickly bubbled to the surface; after all she was still only in her teens. But responsibility soon began to overtake her. Patients from fashionable Cape society soon began to call regularly on her services. In June 1817 her friend Sir Jahleel Brenton sent for her when his wife was dying. Barry was too late to save Lady Brenton but Sir Jahleel retained complete confidence in her ability and continued to consult her himself.

Throughout that year Lord Charles himself seemed eager to advertise Barry's skills. In a letter to the Governor of St Helena, Sir Hudson Lowe, urging him to send his ailing wife on a visit to the Cape with its 'genial' climate, he could not resist adding: 'I have besides here, quite a prodigy as a physician, a Doctor Barry, whose skill has attested wonders since he has been here. Indeed it would be well worthwhile for an invalid to come here solely for the purpose of obtaining his advice.'

When Lord Charles appointed Barry 'Physician to the Governor's Household' at the end of the year he was merely confirming a position that had already been tacitly accepted by the governing class. She had been constantly seen about with the family and had indeed treated them on several occasions. Her new post gave her a cottage in the gracious grounds of Government House and a salary of 600 rix dollars a year (she accepted no fees from her private patients). She was also appointed second member of the Vaccine Institute, which carried a salary of 1200 rix dollars.

However she still remained an officer in uniform – albeit a junior one – with army duties and army pay.

Lord Charles continued to write to his ailing friends recommending his 'prodigy'. In February 1818 Andries Stockenstrom, the Landrost (magistrate) of Graaf Reinet, who had accompanied Lord Charles and his party to meet the Kaffirs, fell ill. Lord Charles (who was something of a hypochondriac) wrote to him 'to entreat that you will not trifle with yourself but that you will repair to Cape Town without delay to have the advantage of Dr Barry's very extraordinary skill'.

To do him justice, Lord Charles did recognize the value of Barry's remarkably advanced methods. Long before scientists understood why wounds turned septic or how disease spread, she insisted on a daily change of linen, frequent dressing of wounds and the most rigorous cleanliness in the sickroom. She made it a rule to clear away any medicines prescribed by other doctors. She campaigned against overcrowding, bad drainage and lack of ventilation in the prisons and hospitals of Cape Town. With more instinct than scientific knowledge, she practised what was, in effect, preventive medicine.

In Guy's Hospital in London where she had trained, the wards were filthy, surgical hygiene was primitive and a professional bug-catcher ranked among the highest-paid members of the staff. It was not until the 1830s that reformers both inside and outside Parliament began to campaign to improve sanitary conditions and to look on public health as a matter of national concern. But during her service at the Cape Dr Barry demanded from individual households and from institutions in Cape Town a standard of sanitation that made some people regard her as an interfering virago.

In September came her first real test as the Governor's physician. Ten days earlier, against her advice, Lord Charles had insisted on visiting the theatre although he had complained of feeling ill. For the next two days he was confined to his home and on the third went out for a short drive in his carriage. He returned in 'a state of great debility' and retired to bed. The gravity of his illness was unexpected and there were soon fears that he was dying. The Colonial Secretary, Lieutenant Colonel Bird, wrote anxiously home to Earl Bathurst at the Colonial Office warning him that the Governor's recovery was regarded as 'extremely precarious'.

On the 29th of September, Colonel Bird was able to report that there were 'some favourable symptoms in his case which Dr Barry tells me is typhus with dysentery'. The Governor's habits of 'great temperance' were in his favour. 'Nevertheless', Colonel Bird added knowledgeably, 'Dr Barry expresses so much apprehension that I cannot delay in making your Lordship acquainted with the state which he now is . . . should an unfavourable turn take place, I shall forthwith despatch the Colonial Schooner [*The Mary*] to England with the tidings . . .'

For four successive nights Lord Charles was delirious from ten in the evening and the schooner was prepared for sea. Barry rarely left his bedside. By October 1st, the crisis had passed, thanks to her vigilance, and Colonel Bird was able to report reassuringly that the Governor had 'rallied a little and was last night without fever . . .' and to add pompously 'considerable hopes are now entertained that he will do well'. Colonel Bird need not have bothered to allay the fears he had aroused in England. Thanks to Barry's intervention the schooner with the news that His Excellency had not twenty-four hours to live had never set sail.

Thirty years later, in a letter to the Governor of Malta, Barry remembered playing a more active part in the drama than the official report suggested:

When I was young, very young, I took on myself the heavy responsibility of differing in opinion from the Inspector-General and three eminent professional men in the case of the Governor, Lord Charles Somerset.

At my earnest request, the Colonial Secretary stopped the dispatches for forty-eight hours and I was left in sole possession of the case; the event justified the difference of opinion – His Lordship survived for many years.

Writing as a Principal Medical Officer, Barry seems to be almost overawed by her youthful daring. Yet at the time she was so sure of herself professionally that, by sheer force of personality she could take over the case and defy the Inspector General. One can see how she must have annoyed her superior officers: perhaps her greatest failing, as far as they were concerned, was that she was so intense. To care so much was hardly good form.

The illness of Lord Charles and Barry's intervention ended the honeymoon period between them. No longer did the Governor write of her with such unrestrained enthusiasm. He was dependent on her, grateful to her. She had saved his life and the life of his daughter. Yet she was a nuisance. She would brook no interference in the sickroom. And she was constantly drawing attention to herself, creating talk and gossip in the mess.

The first note of Lord Charles's irritation with Barry creeps into an account written by Lord Albemarle, a visitor to the Cape. He had heard so much about the extraordinary little doctor that he engineered an opportunity to meet her. Lord Albemarle had himself seated next to Barry at a regimental dinner in the mess. 'In this learned pundit I beheld a beardless lad with an unmistakably Scottish type of countenance, reddish hair and high cheek bones. There was certain effeminacy in his manner which he seemed to be always striving to overcome.' Apparently Barry had recently quarrelled with the Governor who, according to Albemarle, 'was somewhat fanciful about his health'. Dr Barry (the Esculapius, as Albemarle described her) took 'umbrage at something said or done had left his patient to prescribe for himself'. Lord Charles was furious; his prodigy had dared to be insubordinate. 'Dr Barry', the Governor remarked to Albemarle, was 'the most skilful of physicians, most wayward of men'. Another version of that story which circulated in society was that Lord Charles, irritated by something that Barry had said, had picked her up by the scruff of the neck and put her out of the window!

Of course, Barry was never talked about openly as a woman. The idea was too preposterous. Yet hints and innuendoes always hovered. Close observers, like Count de Las Casas and Captain Dillon, were prepared to write down their suspicions and publish them during her lifetime – yet no one dared to challenge her in public.

Everyone in the Colony noticed that Barry reacted with wild fury to any disparaging remark about her size or any slight on her 'masculinity'. There were stories of her flinging wine into fellow officers' faces, slicing off a finger with a sword, lashing out with a whip – or, more credibly, crushing her opponent with her venomous wit.

Another affair, about that time, caused talk for years. She actually fought a duel against Captain Cloete, the Governor's Aide-de-Camp, as Stuart Cloete, the novelist and a descendant of her adversary, can testify. It was, in effect, an affair of the heart.

As her opponent recalled at a regimental dinner years later,

> A buxom lady called to see [Lord Charles] on business of a private nature and they were closeted together for some time. Dr Barry made some disparaging remarks about this: 'Oh, I say Cloete' he sneered, 'that's a nice Dutch filly the Governor has got hold of.' 'Retract your vile expression, you infernal little cad' said I, advancing and pulling the long ugly nose. Barry immediately challenged me and we fought with pistols, fortunately without effect.

The duel was fought under the oaks at Alphen. Absurd as it sounds, Barry was struggling to overcome her jealousy as a woman and translate it into 'manly' actions. Yet however jealous she was it is difficult to understand what possessed her. Since her student days she had struggled to masquerade as a man. By fighting a duel she appeared once again to be courting exposure.

At the time the strain of her situation must have been overwhelming. Hers was not a circumspect nature, despite the burden of secrecy she carried. And there was an even stronger reason. Lord Charles had welcomed her into his family circle. Through him she had been able to lead a carefree existence off-duty for the first time in her life. In the early days at least he had obviously found both her and her situation highly entertaining. As far as she was concerned he was the only man who knew her secret and her family background. Whatever passed between them, it seems clear that he represented father, brother, protector – and even lover. In fact whatever 'normal' emotions she allowed herself to feel for a man were expressed in her relationship with him. Yet as a junior officer of the Governor's household she was forced to affect a deference and a distance in public. Lord Charles's open admiration and respect for her professional ability only made matters worse. He could act out his public role, amused and patronizing, at the expense of his 'most excellent physician'. She, on the other hand, could only drop her guard in private – and even then, one suspects, the Governor grew impatient.

A gentlewoman of the day thus thwarted would have resorted to hysteria, to tears, or to the classic standby of 'delicate health'. Trapped in her role as a man, Barry had no such means of escape. One side of her nature at least must have longed for discovery.

Relatively little is heard of Barry during 1819. Lord Charles was troubled by marauders on the Eastern frontier; settlers were attacked in the spring of the year by about 9000 Bantu and once again the Governor travelled to meet the native chiefs to attempt to stop the raids. This time he travelled by ship with his son Henry, Lt-Colonel Bird and several officers. Dr Barry was not one of the party.

Earlier in the year, Lord Charles had written home to ask for the Prince Regent's permission to return to England on affairs 'of a very urgent nature'. He explained, in a personal note to Lord Bathurst, that he was eager to return because of his great anxiety about his daughter Georgiana's health. He assured the Colonial Secretary that he would be ready to return to the Cape Colony whenever he was asked and merely wanted to convey and settle his daughters.

England at that time faced problems that sound uncannily familiar: unemployment, recession, unrest in the new factories and fear, by the contemporaries of Malthus, of over-population. The Government was anxious to settle colonists in the Second British Empire: men and women emigrated to Canada, Australia and New Zealand, and in January 1820 it was decided to send 5000 settlers to the Cape Colony. As Governor, Lord Charles was asked to postpone his leave until the newcomers had arrived.

Lord Charles could not, or would not, wait. If he neglected to leave it might prove fatal to the health of his daughter, he argued. Before the Governor's departure, a grand ball was given in his honour by the civil and military officers of the Colony. The inside of Society House on the Herrengracht was completely transformed; six doors were removed to accommodate the 400 guests. The lavishly decorated rooms were dotted with arbours of myrtles and flowers and the motto 'Les regrets se mêlent aux plaisirs' (Regrets are mingled with pleasure) displayed everywhere. Officers in brilliant dress, lawyers, civil servants, and their ladies danced quadrilles and country dances through the night.

Curiously, there is no mention that the favourite of the family, Dr Barry, attended. On her army record, written in her own hand, she states that she was 'During the Cholera at Mauritius'. In November 1819 a severe outbreak of cholera had attacked the island and 4000 people had died. But, officially, the news of it did not reach Cape Town until the last days of January 1820 when the Governor of the Bourbon Island sent a report by H.M.S. *Hardy*.

Since the island of Mauritius is 2250 miles from the Cape, a sailing time of at least two to three weeks, it is extremely unlikely that Barry was sent there officially. Was she perhaps on furlough there when the disease broke out? She was eligible for leave – she had worked hard and well for three and a half years – but why did she choose to take it at that moment? Why would Barry want to be absent from the Cape just when Lord Charles was leaving for England? Is it possible that she diplomatically took herself off to have the child which the charwoman, Sophia Bishop, so positively stated she had borne?

4

My Bounden Duty

Once aboard the sloop H.M.S. *Sappho*, Miss Georgiana Somerset, the Governor's eldest unmarried daughter, seems to have recovered with amazing speed. A fortnight after they sailed, the ship docked at St Helena. Sir Hudson Lowe, the Governor of the island and Napoleon's warder, wrote to the Cape that 'Miss Somerset's health has improved on her voyage'. Georgiana's illness may not have been entirely physical in origin. Eighteen months earlier Captain Stirling Glover, a young officer at the Cape, had fallen in love with her and proposed. Lord Charles had forbidden the match on the grounds that the young man's income was 'not adequate to provide her with those indulgences she had always had in her father's house'. So the sea voyage was no accident. But the affair went deep on both sides and, after her father's death, Georgiana married her captain.

'To settle his daughters' was Lord Charles's expressed intention in going home. He himself was soon seen strutting about in London – at the King's birthday celebrations, at levées, receptions and balls given by the aristocracy – and at house parties in the country. The London gossips chattered that he was looking for a wife to settle himself.

A year later, in August 1821, Lord Charles obliged by marrying. He chose a charming and amiable spinster of good family, thirty-two-year-old Lady Mary Poulett, twenty-two years younger than Lord Charles (and ten years older than Barry). A month after his marriage, Lord Charles, his new wife, his two daughters (still unsettled), his servants and a cargo of valuable horses sailed for the Cape aboard the frigate *Hyperion*. They arrived almost two years after their departure, on November 30th, 1821.

Meanwhile, the character of the Colony had changed. Boatloads of English settlers, in small 500-ton vessels, had arrived in the spring of 1820, and they proved a disturbing influence. Moreover they brought disease with them; whooping cough, measles and smallpox. As soon as the boats docked, the settlers were quarantined and then sent off to their settlements on the Eastern Frontier. The pioneer colonists included carpenters, blacksmiths, coopers, farm workers, clergy and doctors, but all found the climate difficult to bear and their own financial situation perilous. It was almost impossible to obtain bank loans. And, as Englishmen, they objected vehemently to the 'unEnglish' laws in the Colony which gave the Governor almost unrestricted power, yet curbed their free speech and deprived them of an independent press.

Since 1818 both Lord Charles, as Governor of the Colony, and the British Government had favoured immigration from England. At home the Government was anxious to relieve over-population and reduce the cost of defending the Colony by settling newcomers on the Eastern Frontier. Government circulars advertising the scheme had omitted Lord Charles's warning that the settlers would have to protect their property from marauding Kaffirs. As a result, they were not at all prepared for the hazards that lay ahead of them.

Economically the Colony was going through a difficult phase, with the value of the rix dollar, the paper money, declining fast. In Lord Charles's absence the Acting Governor, Major-General Sir Rufane Donkin, an ex-Indian Army man, set out to cut costs. He slashed public expenditure on the Governor's residences. He reduced the upkeep of Government House by half and made cuts in outlay on Lord Charles's other three homes: Newlands, the summer residence, the seaside villa at Camp's Bay and the shooting box at Groote Post farm. With settlers so wretchedly poor that they were existing on a diet of fried cabbage and stewed pumpkin, the economies were popular. The Acting Governor also cut back on and altered Lord Charles's plans for policing the frontier. This alteration to the original plans for defence incensed the permanent

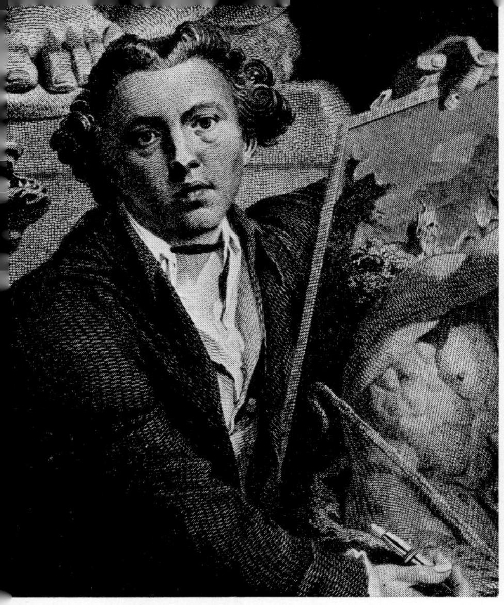

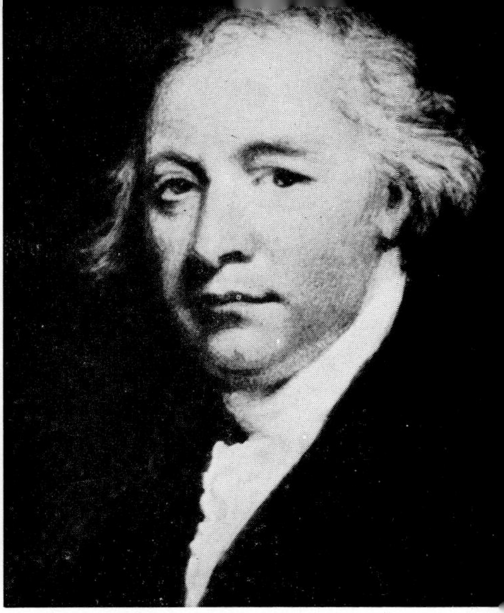

Self-portrait of James Barry, R.A., the Doctor's uncle.

Edmund Burke, the artist's patron, and friend of the Bluestockings.

Lord Buchan, eccentric patron of the artist and his 'nephew'.

General Francisco de Miranda, the Doctor's mentor.

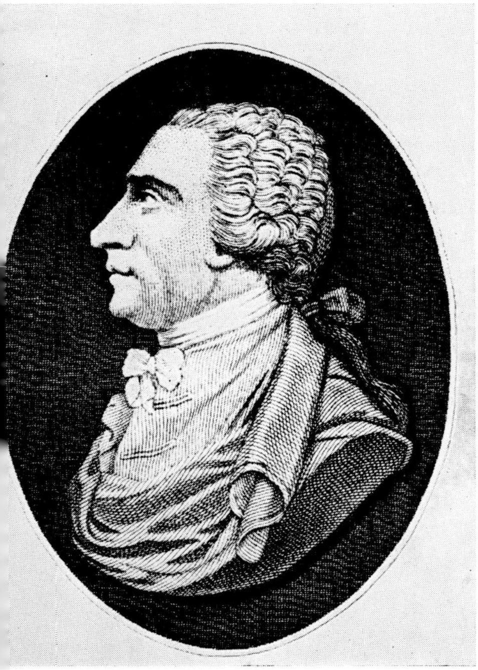

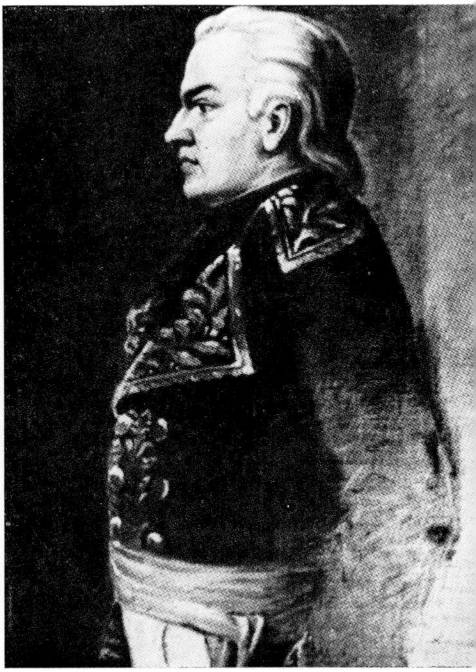

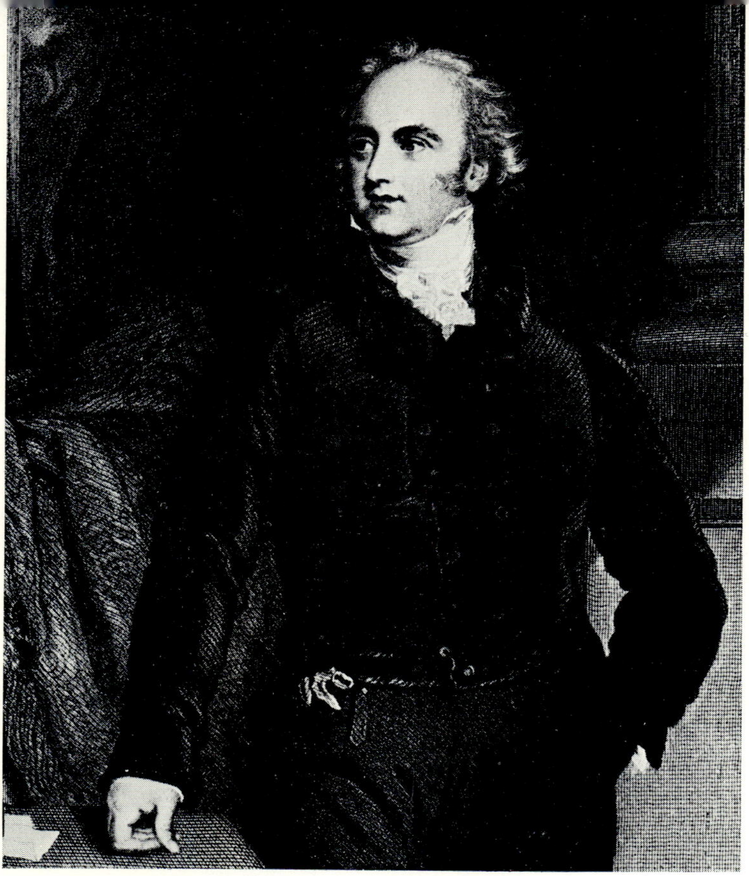

(Above) *Sir Astley Cooper, Professor of Surgery at Guy's Hospital, to whom James Barry was appointed.*

(Below) *Student cards at Edinburgh University where Barry studied from 1810 to 1812.*

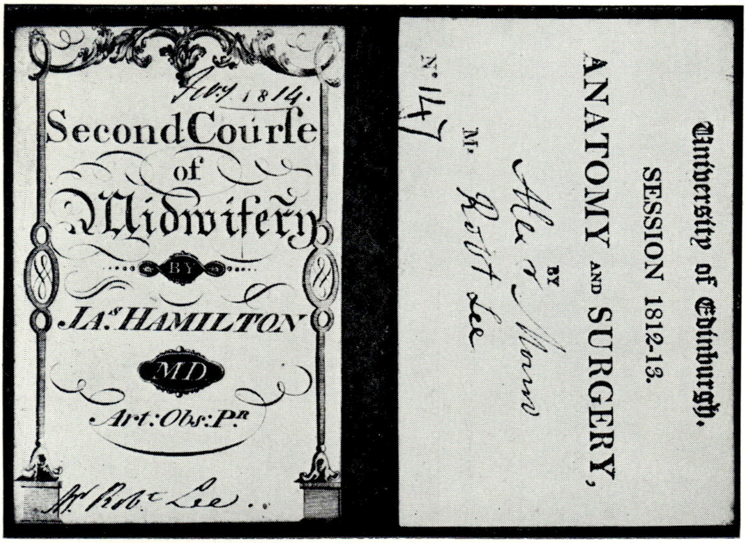

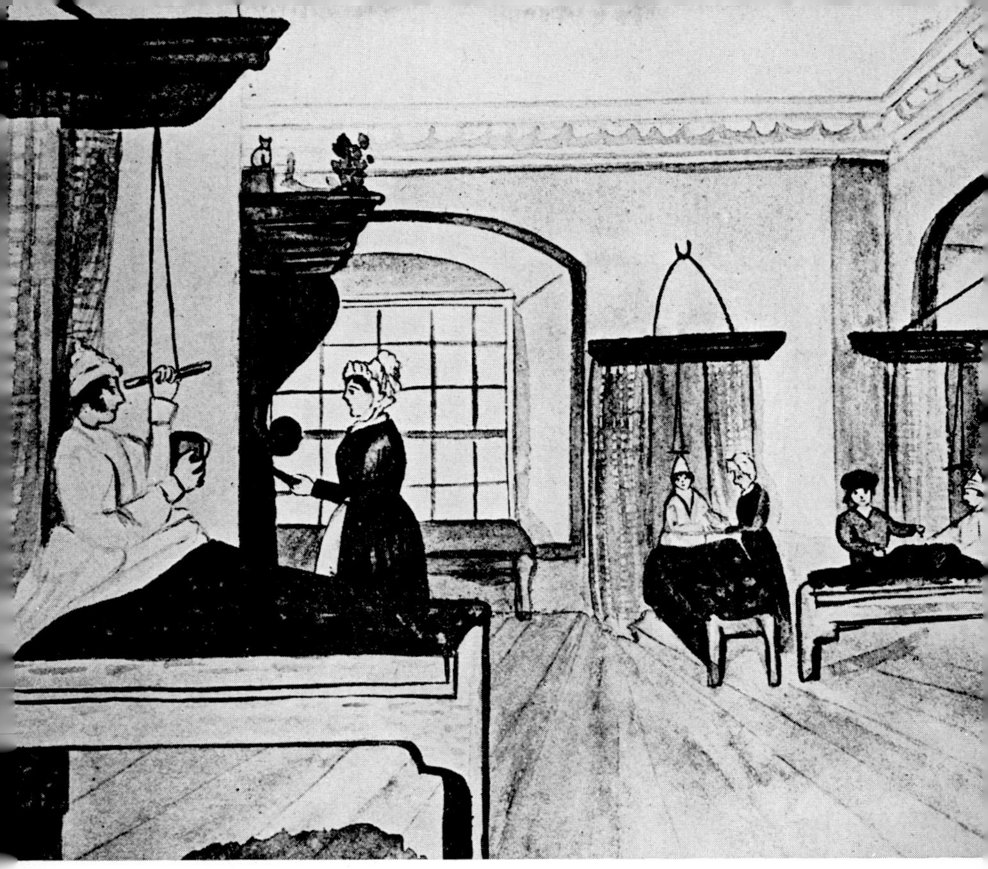

(Above) *Typical hospital ward in the early years of the nineteenth century.*

(Below) *Standard set of instruments issued to army doctors of the period.*

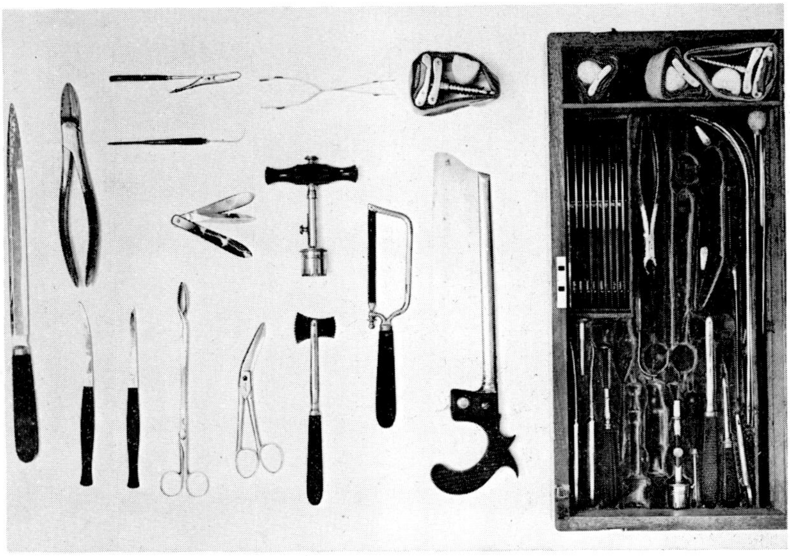

(Right) *Marine Villa, Camps Bay, Cape Town, where the ghost of Dr Barry is supposed to walk.*

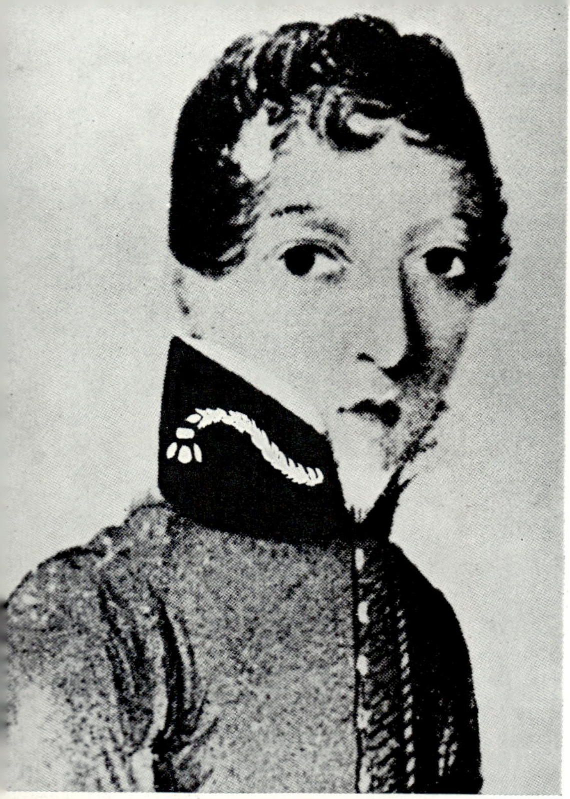

Portrait of Assistant Staff Surgeon Barry on her arrival in Cape Town.

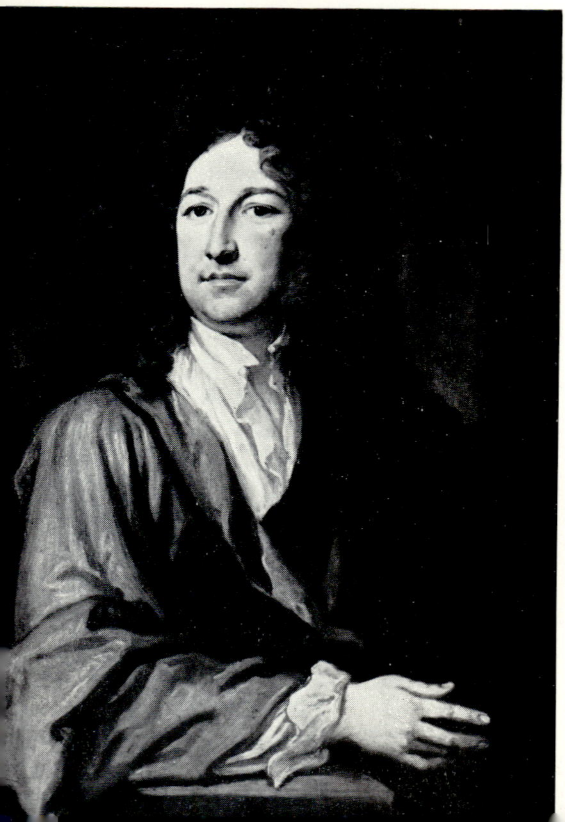

Lord Charles Somerset, Governor of Cape Colony, and Commander-in-Chief of His Majesty's Forces.

(Right) *Examples of conditions that Barry fought against: arbitrary arrest of poor blacks and the chaining of lunatics in their cells.*

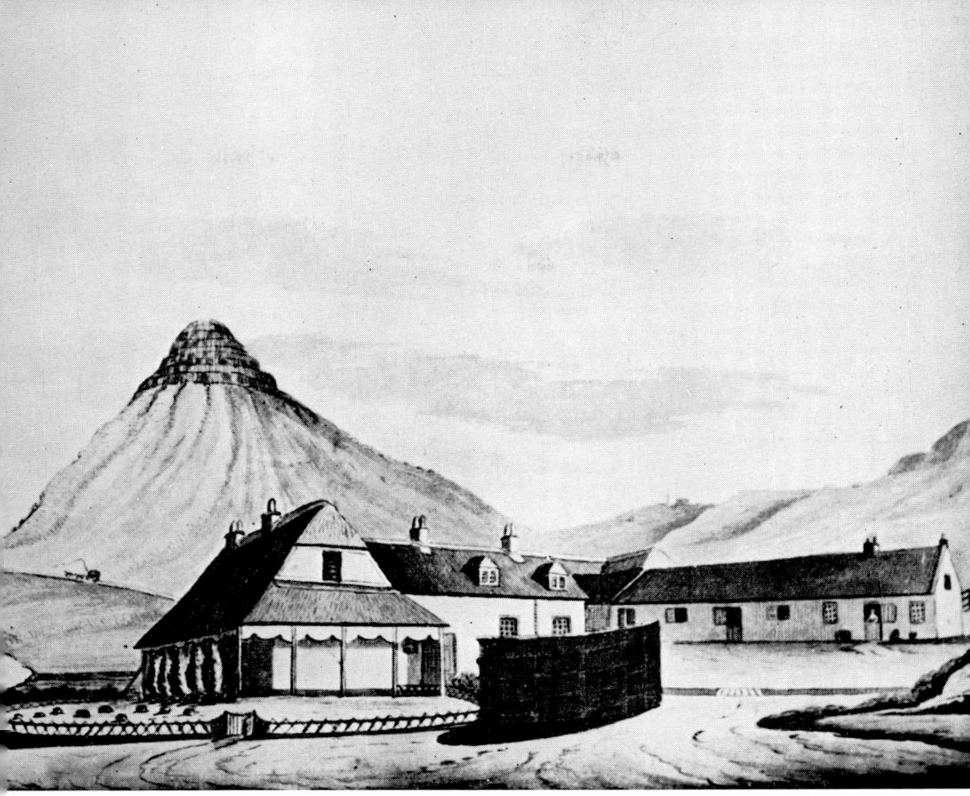

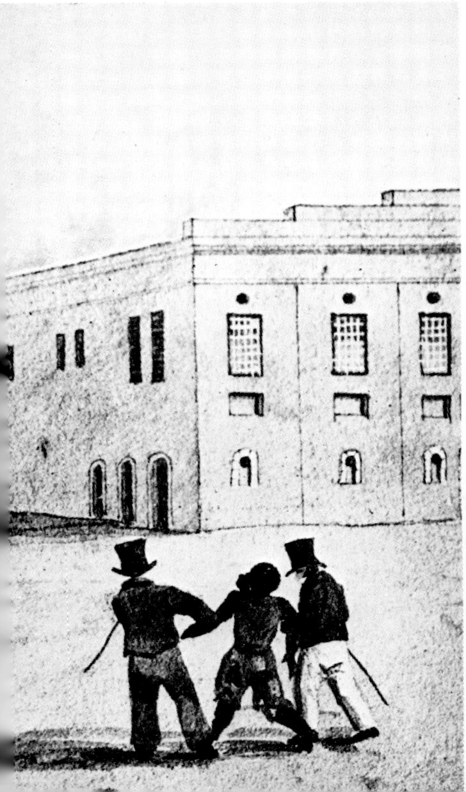

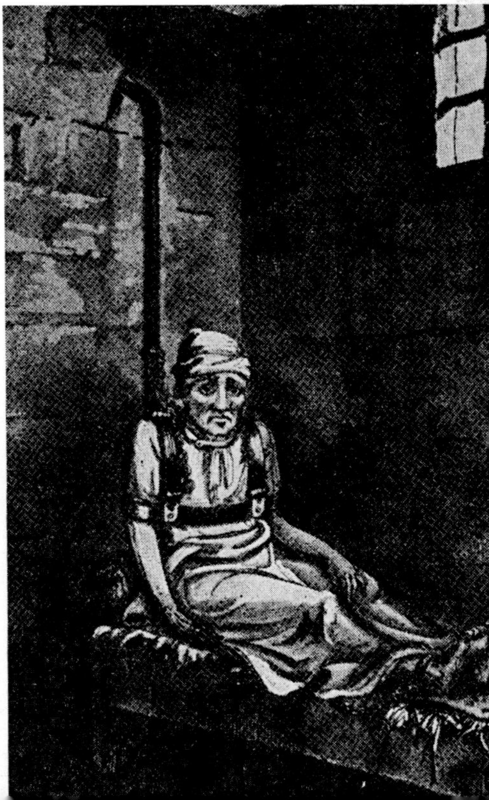

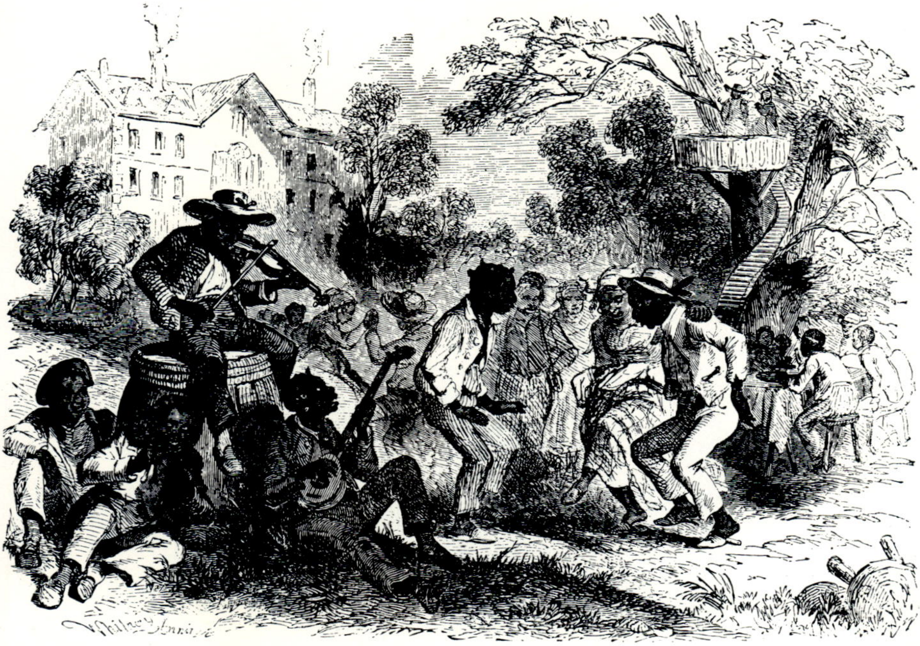

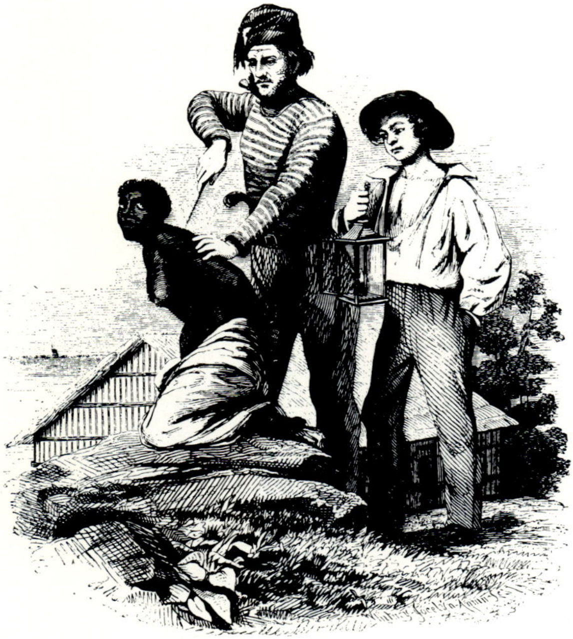

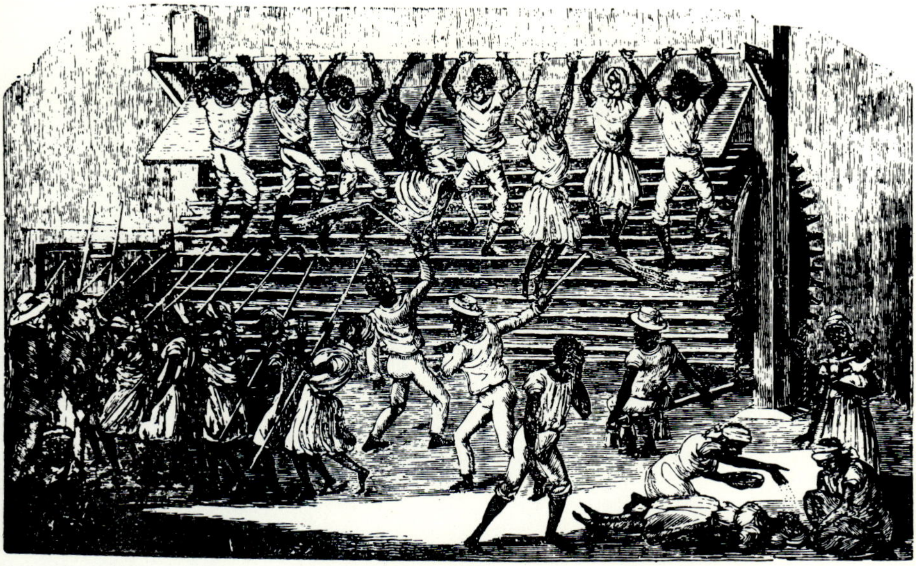

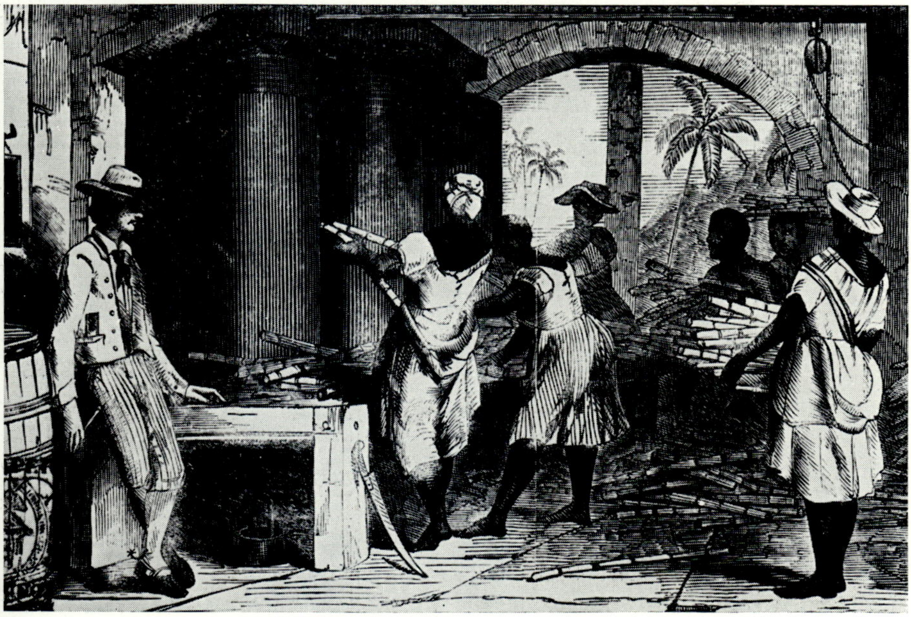

Jamaica, where Dr Barry served from 1831 to 1835. When a festival turned into a riot, Barry was appalled at the harsh treatment of the blacks and shocked at the dreadful conditions on the plantations.

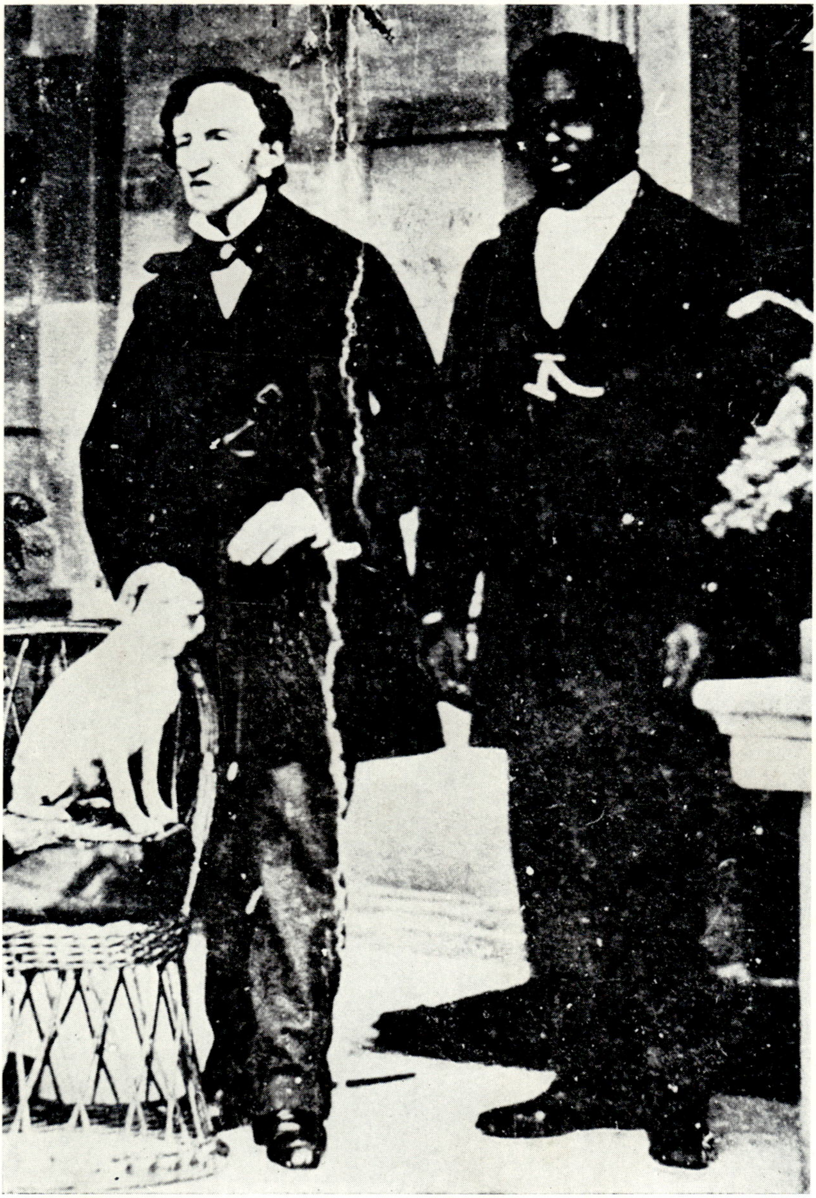

A rare photograph of Dr Barry taken in Jamaica circa 1860. As usual, she is accompanied by her poodle, Psyche, and a black servant.

Governor and aroused criticism at home. Sir Rufane also decided on a new site for a township at Bathurst. In January 1820 troops moved in to protect the settlers, a Commissariat was established and work begun on public buildings. The pioneers invested considerable sums in the construction of the town. However, two years later Lord Charles was to change the site of the town, with the result that the anticipated boom never materialized and the angry settlers lost their money.

Napoleon's presence at St Helena had created a temporary prosperity at the Cape, since foodstuffs and wine were sent to the island to supply the large establishment that had grown up around the former Emperor. Napoleon was ill in December 1820 and Sir Hudson Lowe wrote to Earl Bathurst, uncertain as to whether the illness was real or feigned. Earl Bathurst recommended sending to the Cape for help, 'where there was a doctor with a great reputation'. But before the reply could reach St Helena, Napoleon died. Dr Barry, to whom, of course, the noble Earl was referring, narrowly missed the chance to treat Napoleon.

During the years of Lord Charles's absence little is known of Dr Barry. She presented several of her books, bearing her own book-plate, to the new public library which opened in January 1822. The Library Committee also consulted her about the merits of various medical books. In May 1821, perhaps as a result of Sir Rufane Donkin's economy drive, Assistant Surgeon James Barry was placed by general order on half-pay – a not unreasonable directive. She was earning 600 rix dollars a year as the Governor's personal physician (the rix dollar by then had slumped in value to about one shilling and ninepence) in addition to her salary as a member of the Vaccine Institute.

When Lord Charles arrived back at the Cape on the afternoon of November 30th, 1821, a small boarding party of three officers – Captain Henry Somerset (Lord Charles's son), Major Josiah Cloete (Barry's ex-duelling opponent) and Dr James Barry – went aboard to welcome him.

Barry must have found it hard to accept the new situation but she fought down her feelings in order to greet the Governor and his party as a loyal member of his staff. All through her life her attachment to Charles Somerset was undoubtedly her most important human contact and it must have been painful for her to see him as a married man. The Governor was not an imaginative man. He was not troubled about Barry's feelings. His main concern was to learn exactly what had been happening in the Colony during his absence. He was anxious to uphold his position and reassert his authority. The story of the 'misdeeds' of Sir Rufane Donkin poured out by the loyal trio infuriated him. He was particularly put out by the quarrel that the Acting Governor had 'dared' to pick with his son Henry Somerset.

Sir Rufane had removed some high-bred Spanish mules belonging to Lord Charles from Newlands where they had been grazing at the public expense. Captain Henry Somerset was furious and, when they met on the road one day, demanded their return. Sir Rufane then shook his horsewhip at the Governor's son and barred him from coming to Cape Town.

Lord Charles had a somewhat exaggerated sense of family loyalty. 'No one has ever embroiled himself with anyone of my family without regretting it', he once told an official – and since Henry Somerset was a rather hot-headed officer and an unpopular magistrate, he often landed his father in trouble. This time, however, the 'trouble' was to produce political repercussions of a new, and unexpectedly serious, nature.

When a staff officer arrived aboard the frigate with a message from Sir Rufane Donkin inviting the party to dinner at Government House, he was sent back with word that Lord Charles would be dining on board.

At six o'clock the next morning, Sir Rufane finished his breakfast and went down to the beach to welcome the Governor. While he was out, Lord Charles walked into Government House and, despite his offer to see the Acting Governor 'if Sir R. Donkin has any official communications to make', the two administrators never met. Sir Rufane returned aggrieved to England to report on the state of affairs in the Colony and gather support for a counter-attack. In the meantime anyone who had shown the least civility to the Acting Governor was suspect as far as Lord Charles was concerned.

From now on Lord Charles chose to live at Newlands, five miles outside Cape Town. Whether this was because the climate suited his new bride (now pregnant), or whether he wanted to distance himself from his household physician, is uncertain. But he did keep Barry busy. In February 1822 she was a member of a board appointed to consider the question of effective quarantine for ships coming in from nearby colonies. Rigorous methods were employed. Bedding and clothes were hung in the rigging and aired for days, and foul linen was dipped in the sea, wrung out and aired before being sent ashore to be washed.

In March 1822 Dr James Barry received her real chance. Dr Robb, the Colonial Medical Inspector, resigned and Barry was offered the post at a salary of 2400 rix dollars (about £177) a year. Lord Charles urged her to accept and leave the Army; he gave her to understand that it was to be a permanent appointment. No doubt he felt that civilian office was more befitting. The post of Colonial Medical Inspector carried considerable authority. Until September 1821 the practice of medicine at the Cape had been governed by a Medical Board, consisting of a group of doctors. As part of his economy drive, Sir Rufane had abolished the board and vested its authority in a single doctor.

Barry accepted the job, but decided to stay on in the Army as Assistant Surgeon on half-pay – regarded in those days as a kind of retainer for officers. As it turned out this was to prove the wisest decision of her career.

However her new responsibilities underlined the anomaly of her position. As a twenty-three-year-old Assistant Staff Surgeon, she was a very junior officer, but her post as Colonial Medical Inspector entitled her to a secretary, an office and a great deal of authority. The Colonial Medical Inspector's principal duties were to inspect all drugs imported into the Colony, to grant licences to doctors, apothecaries and accoucheurs (male midwives) and to supervise the practice of medicine. When Barry took over standards were lax: she grappled immediately with her task and widened its scope.

She was never quite at home with bureaucracy. On her appointment she applied to the Colonial Secretary for stationery – fifty quills, a blotting case, four quires of foolscap, two quires of letter paper, a quire of blotting paper and two pencils – the normal supply for the job and one which her predecessor Dr Robb had received free. She did not get it. And there were other petty irritations. The Post Office refused to deliver free letters to her on the grounds that Mr Murray, a Staff Surgeon and senior to her, was the person entitled to the privilege. She also had to press her claim to receive *The*

Courant, the Government Gazette, which she needed to scan the advertisements of the sale of medicines. Her office entitled her to all these privileges. Was it her youth, her manner or the instinctive recognition that she was an outsider that caused others to place so many minor obstructions in her path?

But petty obstacles did not stop her – indeed almost nothing could stop her from doing what she saw as her duty. Not even Lord Charles could do that. Within days of assuming office, Barry was laying down the law about how physicians, surgeons, apothecaries and accoucheurs were to behave professionally. In the past, as Barry graphically explained, laws had been allowed to lapse and abuse had crept in. 'Apothecaries were practising medicine, physicians were keeping shop and shopkeepers were selling drugs.' She cracked down hard. 'To my certain knowledge', she wrote, 'many persons have been poisoned by patent medicines given improperly.' Since these quacks and pedlars did not understand the nature of the medicines they were selling, they could not prescribe an antidote. Hence the mischief.

She told a district surgeon in the interior that arsenic and opium (classified as dangerous drugs today) should not be dispensed without the sanction of a qualified doctor. In the country areas district surgeons acted as apothecaries and accoucheurs, sometimes without any qualifications at all. They could prescribe castor oil, emetics and other household medicines, she allowed; but no apothecary was to practise as physician, surgeon or accoucheur on pain of having his licence removed. Although, she added, with (female?) commonsense, if there was an emergency, then the district surgeon or apothecary was not prevented from giving first aid!

District surgeons were to act as apothecaries and to make up the prescriptions which Barry ordered. They could not refuse night calls and must attend police, prisoners, convicts and paupers in their district, free of charge. The local authorities, she decided, were to foot the bill.

But her reforms did not stop there. One of her most important measures was to introduce a systematic plan for vaccination against smallpox throughout the Colony almost twenty years before such a measure was introduced in England.

She made herself unpopular by personally inspecting shops

to make sure her orders were carried out. At Bianchi's in Plein Street, Cape Town, one customer had died and several were dangerously ill because of improper sales. The proprietor was selling medicines without a licence. Dr Liesching, the prison doctor, kept a leading apothecary's shop and supplied the prison with drugs from it (a very convenient arrangement).

True to her principles even when it put her own career at risk, she ordered several hundredweight of drugs imported by Dr Liesching, including four hundredweight of Epsom salts and twenty-nine pounds of camphor, to be destroyed because they were damaged. Irregularities were constantly drawn to her notice. A horse doctor in the district of Bathurst was drawing teeth, treating sore legs and dislocated limbs!

Although she was blamed, all through her career, for her apparent officiousness, she showed considerable tact when a dispute arose which did not concern the health and wellbeing of the patient. If, for example, it was a question of an account, of money between patient and doctor, Barry was loath to act officially. Better, she felt, 'if the affair was arranged amiably'.

She showed an astonishingly mature grasp of administration in those early years. She rationalized fees for the medical profession, taking into account the depreciation of the rix dollar, and persuaded the Governor to renew the Proclamation for Regulating Medical Practice. And as for her measures against the illegal sale of drugs, eighteen months after she took office, she could report that the regulations had been strict enough

> to alarm and deter Pedlars and Quacks and all Pretenders to medicine, from selling medicines and practising to the utter destruction of the poor Patients, as well as to the manifest injury of the educated Practioner, who as long as such Persons were permitted to puff off their own wonderful abilities and the supernatural Excellencies of their drugs . . . it was impossible for the honest practitioner to obtain even his daily bread by his profession.

A professional to her fingertips, she believed that it was better in all cases 'to be without advice than to have bad advice whether in Lay or Physic'.

It must have seemed to other officials, used to the complacency of colonial administration, that Dr Barry had an exaggerated sense of her responsibilities. When she became Colonial

Medical Inspector, she took on duties that no one before her had even dreamt of, *and* persuaded Lord Charles that he had asked her to perform them! It was the plight of the most wretched in the Colony that concerned her: the convicts, the paupers, the lunatics and the lepers.

When Barry took office, rumours were reaching the capital that the lepers in the colony at Swellendam were so neglected and starving that they were escaping to find food. Barry set out to discover the truth for herself. To reach the leper colony she had to make an arduous journey of seventy or eighty miles across the mountains. On October 25th, 1822, she rode on horseback to conduct a conference at 'Heaven and Earth'. She invited the Rev. Dr Thom, the Religious Instructor, Dr O'Flinn from Stellenbosch and the Field Cornet to meet her and review the position. But it was to the lepers that Barry primarily addressed herself.

She explained to them that she was the Governor's messenger, sent to investigate their complaints. Those who could stand showed her their emaciated bodies, barely covered by the filthy rags they wore. In the hospital there were four lepers unable to move: one lay on a dirty stretcher, the rest on the ground. The rest of the wretched, unsightly men and women were hungry and maltreated. They were made to work in the garden, no matter how ill they felt, and punished if they slacked.

'Nothing', Barry wrote, appalled, 'could excel the misery of the 120 lepers squalid and wretched beyond description. I found the Medical Department neglected. The doctor seemed to take not the slightest interest in the poor people entrusted to his care.'

The land allotted to the leper institution was in beautiful spacious grounds, but the lepers themselves occupied only a small part of them. In a kraal belonging to the colony Barry found three cows originally intended to supplement the lepers' meagre diet, but now taken from them! In the Governor's name she immediately ordered an increase in the lepers' rations and set about improving their standards of medicine, hygiene and comfort.

The staff had ready excuses. The doctor complained that he was badly paid, had difficulty in making the journey, and that riding over rough roads affected his health. It transpired that in bad weather he did not come at all. The Religious Instructor lived a four-hour horseback journey from the colony. And the steward on the spot grumbled that he was bullied and made to do all the doctor's work and yet only allowed to administer 'a dose of salts' or apply blue-stone to the wounds of the lepers.

Barry was not concerned with excuses. It was the lepers' misery that stung her into action. With her usual vigour she reported very fully to Lord Charles. Through the gossips in the Government's clerical department her vivid accounts of suffering and injustice – somehow too personal to be ignored – touched the public conscience.

The Governor seems to have accepted her views, amused, tolerant, even touched by her concern. She suggested that lepers who were fit should be paid for doing light work 'with a little wine, a few shillings or some tobacco or coffee so that they would cheerfully contribute to cultivate the soil to increase their own comforts'. To a group of wretches, black, destitute, ill and outcast, she brought the comfort that somebody in authority cared about their condition.

As a physician to the leading members of Cape society she was often consulted privately. She was notorious for her extraordinary methods; almost every old family in Cape Town had a tale to tell about her. Late one night, she was called in to a fine old homestead, five miles from the town, where a Mrs Cloete was lying apparently dangerously ill with pneumonia. She arrived at the house in her horse and buggy and the weeping members of the family solemnly conducted her to the sickroom. As soon as she entered the bedroom, a blast of hot air almost overcame her. She stamped her foot on the ground, rushed to the window and flung it open. Next she went to the patient's four-poster bed and tore the curtains apart in a frenzy. Then she rounded on the startled and mournful relatives and gave them the telling off of their lives. Within minutes she stormed out of the room, ordering only that the bedroom should be kept thoroughly aired.

The patient was shocked back to health and remained an admirer of Dr Barry. Since she insisted that as a Government officer she could not accept payment, Mrs Cloete chose two fine black horses from her stud farm and sent them up to the Castle for the doctor's use. Every year, for as long as Barry remained in Cape Town, a wagonload of forage from her grateful patient was delivered to her.

The contrast between the life of the governing class, with their sumptuous dinners, their hunting, shooting and racing, and the plight of the wretched lepers could not fail to scar a nature like hers. In 1822 high society at the Cape, led by Lord Charles and his lady, acknowledged the benefits of sea-bathing, thanks to Barry's influence – but she had already ordered that the lepers too should enjoy regular and healthy immersions. A year later the Moravian missionary Brother Leitner complained that because of the sea-bathing 'there were but few hearers at our worship and we were obliged to put off Holy Communion'.

The missionary's main aim was to convert the lepers and he resented Barry's interference. Barry herself was devout, but her priority was healing. And she was convinced that medicine alone would not benefit the lepers. In her view cleanliness and exercise were imperative. However, even she admitted that most of the lepers, prize Negroes or Hottentots, worked by their masters until they looked too repulsive to use, were beyond help. To the remote, aristocratic circles Barry moved in, her concern must have seemed absurd in the extreme. She dined out, she lived the life of an important official, she appeared to be one of the most lively and well-informed 'bachelors' of the Colony. To spend a sixteen-hour day trying to improve the conditions of blacks – and lepers to boot! – must have seemed absolutely ridiculous. Certainly Lord Charles could not understand her behaviour. He described her to one official as 'the greatest physician I have ever met', but 'absurd in everything else'. Was the passion she brought to her work an overcompensation for a lonely, an impossible life?

To the lepers in 'Heaven and Earth' (some might have called it hell) it did not matter. She cared. She came. In March 1823 she left Cape Town at four in the morning. After a three-hour ride the party was held up at the far side of the river by a pole at the landing place. It was too early for the ferryman! Despite the danger to herself and her party she plunged in and swam across the river on horseback, determined to reach the leper colony in good time. This time she was pleased to find the patients were looking healthier and cleaner. They seemed more contented with the missionary and his wife.

More practical suggestions followed her visit. The diet of the lepers was to consist of rice, milk and coffee with vegetables when possible. 'If His Excellency the Governor should think fit', she added rather wistfully in her report 'it would greatly benefit the lepers if some vegetable seeds and a few vine slips or even some fruit trees were sent up for their use.'

For the lepers, Barry considered that a soldier's ration was 'medically adequate'. But from a human point of view she added, 'as a keen appetite seems almost part of the disease I should by no means recommend these poor people being deprived of their pound of mutton or their bread'. 'Soup should always be insisted on', she recommended, since there were so many women and children as well as invalids in the Colony. She wanted two or three cooks, two nurses to keep the hospital clean and look at, or even dress, the wounds. 'If His Excellency approve these remarks and continue the institution under my charge, I shall . . . consider what further in a Professional point of view might be done for the benefit of that Institution.'

His Excellency did approve them. To do him credit he seems to have appreciated the improvements Barry made. But her reforms, and the measures needed to put them into practice, were expensive. She wanted to visit the leper colony again in May 1823, but the cost to the public of providing horses was considered too great. When she was allowed to return in June, what she found frustrated and angered her. Most of the lepers were nearly naked and 'the person who has the contract (for clothing) declares that he cannot deliver them within two months'. And, despite her 'continual and earnest remonstrances to the contrary', the patients were given a ration of meal instead of bread.

Barry noticed a number of fine, healthy children aged between two and fifteen still free of the disease, and pleaded for them. She diplomatically suggested that it would save the Government money if the children were removed from the colony:

> Should it meet with the approbation of Lord Charles to remove these children from the institution and apprentice them out . . . it would be a great measure to check the spreading and propagation of this loathsome disease, which has been hitherto so rapidly increasing and not only diminish the Government Expense but also the children themselves would be rendered useful members of society.

In the face of Barry's searing compassion, the Governor had little choice.

A legend exists in the capital that Barry herself had a leper son whom she kept hidden in a large walled garden in the Oranjezicht, a suburb of Cape Town, on the slopes of Table Mountain. It would have been in character for her to adopt one of the children she found growing up in the squalor of 'Heaven and Earth'. And, unless she really had a child of her own (and another legend suggests that her own son died very young), it would have been somebody to love, apart from Psyche (she always had a poodle called Psyche), and the remote Lord Charles, now married and living at Newlands.

One almost gets the impression that she was seeking Lord Charles's approval in the constant battery of reports that she sent him. But apart from her one-woman crusade to reform conditions in the leper colony, her efforts to improve the town prison (or Tronk), Robben Island (where long-term convicts were sent), and the civilian Somerset Hospital, were beginning to cause a stir among the discontented English settlers. James Barry was proving an embarrassment to the Governor.

The Somerset Hospital was founded in 1818 by an Englishman, Samuel Bailey, a naval surgeon who had served at Waterloo. He had paid for the hospital out of his own pocket for four years, but by the time Barry took charge of the health of the civilians of the Colony, Dr Bailey could no longer afford the upkeep of the hospital. He had sold it to the municipality, and the worthy burghers had allowed the hospital to deteriorate badly.

With Mr McCarthy, the Colonial Paymaster, Barry visited the hospital and reported on the section devoted to lunatics. 'Fifteen individuals . . . and the whole establishment void of cleanliness, order or professional care.' She recommended that a patient with a head injury needing attention be transferred to the Military Hospital; she reported that a woman, a native of Bourbon named Francina, was 'as sane as most people and by no means a subject for a lunatic hospital'. An old woman, said to be over 100 years old, in her second childhood, needed, she observed, not the miseries, but even in the most moderate way, the necessities of life. The poor creature had neither bed nor blanket. Two others, a carpenter working at his trade and another man she considered sane, were recommended for discharge. 'The other ten are lunatics but they require also a little attention', she added laconically.

This was an outrageously modern conclusion in the 1820s, for in England the public's attitude towards lunatics was barbaric. A committee, appointed in 1815 to investigate conditions in 'madhouses', discovered 'grave abuses': unaccounted-for deaths among patients; shortage of staff and consequently excessive use of the straitjacket or the chains and leg irons. The public still flocked to Bedlam to watch the antics of the insane, where, as in other madhouses, the wretched inmates were purged, bled, blistered, forced to vomit, knocked down and plunged in cold baths. In Bethnal Green a woman patient was housed in a former pigsty. It was not until 1828 that a bill was passed appointing fifteen Commissioners in the Metropolitan district to visit homes for the insane.

Five years before and 6000 miles away Dr Barry was advocating far more drastic reforms. Her disconcerting approach was reflected not only in her views but in her direct and cutting style of writing. She disturbed the worthy townspeople and the cautious civil servants – and she would not give up. Again and again she filed complaints against the Somerset Hospital where the lunatics had no beds or bedding. 'The wards are as dirty as the patients', she wrote. 'Nothing but a general reform could improve the place which does not deserve to be dignified with the title of Hospital.'

With her colleagues, however, she was honest and fair-minded, if – to them – something of a prig. When Dr Robert Shand (a qualified doctor from Aberdeen) reported that a slave had died from a flogging with the birch, the district surgeon, Dr Tardieux, examined the body a week later and tried to whitewash the evidence. He pronounced that the slave, a heavy eater, had died from '*bulimih*' (abnormal hunger and over-eating which causes occasional fainting). Barry upheld Dr Shand's verdict, and added acidly that Tardieux had not dissected the body and his assertion that bruises could not cause death was not only false and mischievous, but ignorant in the extreme.

In many unspectacular ways she was an innovator. When an epidemic broke out she not only summoned her colleagues and gave explicit instructions about treatment, hygiene and diet, she also published advice to the public on how to recognize and treat measles, smallpox and plague, as well as instructions on suitable foods for the sick and convalescent. Her written advice was the beginning of home nursing in South Africa.

But she is remembered principally for the storms and the scandal. By the time she had been in office for a year she was in conflict with the merchants who imported patent medicines, with the worthy burghers who ran the town hospital, and with some of the town's most well-known physicians (a rather sour note in the Cape Medical Society earlier recorded that although army medical officers were frequently consulted by their civilian colleagues, the courtesy was never reciprocated). She was also battling with the missionary at the leper colony, who was still smarting under her criticism.

Brother Leitner believed he was in sole charge of the colony. He resented Barry's interference and even her medical directions. He complained that medicines *he* had ordered had directions written on them 'probably by Dr Barry'. The set of rules that Barry had laid down annoyed him too. They were sound and practical, calling for strict attention to the personal cleanliness of the lepers – change of bedding and clothing, and bathing, at least twice a week (once a day for the children). As to medical care, she had ordered that the sores should be washed twice daily with tar water and dressed with tar paste; and that old plasters should be thrown away. Bowels were to be attended to and cases of venereal disease separated from the rest. Very bad cases of leprosy were to be isolated also, and wine given to the sick. In her own words, 'Good order must be preserved but no cruelty nor deprivation of food must ever be resorted to . . . They must be considered not as convicts but as unfortunates.' School and church were to be encouraged and 'as much industry as possible'.

Barry invariably laid down the law not only about hygiene and diet but also about attitudes to patients, a practice that put her at least a century ahead of her time. But she was bossy and she infuriated Brother Leitner, who considered that she was undermining his authority. The Governor had given him to understand that he could always rely on official support.

Barry ordered the missionary to report to her on the patients' health every week, and warned that her visits would be frequent. Leitner objected to the injunction and to Barry's assumption of authority. He even threatened to resign rather than carry on under her.

By the close of 1823 Barry's campaign to improve conditions for the outcasts of the Colony had met with some success. But her impatience for reform was bringing her increasingly into conflict with the most powerful forces in Cape society. She was soon to learn that a medical administrator needed to act with diplomacy as well as professional integrity.

5

'Honi Soit . . .'

Eighteen-twenty-four was a year of trouble. The year began badly with newspapers in England, the *Morning Chronicle* and *The Times*, attacking the Cape Government. The troubles of the English settlers with their four failed harvests (rust, a hitherto unknown disease, had attacked the wheat crop), their land heavily mortgaged, bank loans an impossibility and their cattle and farm instruments frequently stolen by raiding Kaffirs, caused anxiety at home. Meetings were held in the City of London about the wretched state of the settlers.

Disquiet in England about the settlers' plight prompted Parliament to instruct a Commission of Inquiry, appointed primarily to reform Colonial Government in Ceylon and Mauritius, to include a visit to the Cape in their itinerary. The two Commissioners, Mr J. T. Bigge, a former judge, and Major Colebrooke, landed at Simonstown in July 1823. Ironically both Dr Barry and Lord Charles were closely connected with the anti-slavery lobby responsible for the Commissioners' visit. Wilberforce, who introduced the debate on 'Slavery at the Cape of Good Hope', was a close friend of the Duchess of Beaufort, Lord Charles's mother, and also of Sir Jahleel Brenton, Dr Barry's ally. At the Cape, the Commissioners were briefed to introduce the English language into the Courts and to change the legal system gradually so that it would conform to the principles of British justice, 'more immediately with regard to the British Community'. They were soon bombarded with complaints about the administration.

The settlers, it was claimed, were 'sinking into a state of

degradation, indolence, destitution and despair'. After six months of campaigning, a free newspaper, the *South African Commercial Advertiser*, had been established which could air the grievances of the new English middle class, leading settlers in a colony which, as one said, 'dreaded political debate'. As a senior civil servant Barry was inevitably involved. Suspicion of corruption among officials, misappropriation of funds and property, hitherto barely conceivable, was creeping into the press. The Collector of Customs, a Mr Blair, was attacked in a 'memorial' to Lord Charles for abusing his authority in distributing prize Negroes (slaves imported into the Colony illegally). He was, it was alleged, apprenticing the Negroes to his creditors. Instead of forwarding the memorandum to the Treasury, Lord Charles prosecuted its author for 'defamation of a public servant'. The Governor's instinctive response to criticism was to suppress it.

The bad blood between Lord Charles Somerset and Sir Rufane Donkin (the Acting Governor in the years 1820–1) had meant that decisions taken by him were reversed by Lord Charles. The siting of Bathurst, for example, had been changed to Grahamstown, with great hardship to the settlers. Soon Lord Charles engineered the dismissal of his former Secretary, Colonel Bird, who had been friendly to Sir Rufane Donkin after the two Governors quarrelled. But not all Lord Charles's actions were so partisan; he reversed a number of land grants made by his deputy – and for once the Government at home upheld his decision without demur.

Since his second marriage in 1821 and the subsequent removal of the influence of the young and idealistic Dr Barry, Lord Charles was less often to be seen away from his estate. He seemed to have become a changed man. He had taken over a colony ruled by Roman Dutch Law, where the Governor was absolute dictator. Then the arrival of the English settlers with their deep-rooted love of freedom had called for change and the two Commissioners of Inquiry were attempting to introduce a system of government more palatable to the Englishman. But Lord Charles, related by blood or marriage to all the great families of England, was scarcely the man to countenance change. He ruled the Colony with the feudalism and paternalism of a Tory squire and treated the territory as if it were his own estate. He was, however, influenced by his mother's opposition to slavery and his attitude to the slaves at the Cape was comparatively enlightened. He also permitted – and perhaps showed an uncomfortable sympathy with – Barry's agitation for reform. However he could not stomach even the suggestion that his absolute authority should be undermined.

In all the ferment Barry was in favour of the free press (how, with her upbringing, could she be other?) Her campaign for humane conditions for prisoners and paupers, lunatics and convicts, was unwittingly helping to unseat the Governor. She rather naïvely believed that her crusade was against the *local* authorities and felt it her 'bounden duty' to inform the Governor of all the injustices she uncovered.

In the course of the crusade she made many enemies. The 'ignorant and mercenary' merchants and shopkeepers (as she termed them) hated her. These importers of patent medicines and 'wonder' cures had lost a lot of money through her rigorous inspection of their wares, and early in 1824 fifty-one of them banded together to protest against her in a memorandum to the Governor. They had invested large sums of money in patent medicines, they protested, 'on the faith of being allowed to sell said medicines sanctioned by His Majesty's Royal Letters Patent and also by immemorial usage and custom'. They objected, so they claimed, not so much to the inspection itself, as to the power vested in one individual, 'however respectable that individual may be and on which subject your Memorialists do not intend by these observations to cast the least shadow of a reflection'! And, they argued, the Colonial Medical Inspector could not 'inspect' patent medicines because he did not know their composition.

'Balsam of Lilley', 'Wonderful Essence', 'Red Powder', and so on, could cause no mischief, they claimed. Indeed, chorused the memorialists, they could cite cases of where patients had recovered by using these medicines long after 'a regular practitioner has given over the patient'. On the 24th of May the Colonial Secretary forwarded the memorandum to Dr Barry. Four days later she wrote what was, for her, a very restrained reply. She pointed out that the power to inspect drugs had been vested in one individual for eleven years, although not exercised; that, as Colonial Medical Inspector, she did not attempt to analyse the drugs, merely to make sure that they answered their description and were not damaged in passage. 'Pedlars and hawkers of drugs do more real injury to the inhabitants than the most virulent diseases themselves', she added. 'Moreover a regularly educated man cannot with justice to himself and the community settle in the interior when Quacks and quack medicine are first resorted to.' And, she added coolly, if the merchants wished to employ other medical men to attend the inspection, they were free to do so.

It was a triumph for Barry. Forewarned of the merchants' attack she convened a meeting of leading physicians, surgeons, apothecaries, druggists and chemists, at her house on the 21st April. The medical men sent a counter-memorandum to Lord Charles, urging the need for inspection of patent medicines, the desirability of their sale by professional men who knew what they were selling, and suggesting that hawkers and pedlars in country villages should be obliged to buy their medicines from the country surgeon or from the regular apothecaries in Cape Town. The pedlars could then be told of the proper use of the drugs. This measure would guard the public from 'dangerous and spurious' medicine.

For Barry, the year must have seemed like a succession of battles. Charles Fredrik Liesching, the prison doctor's son, was himself pressing Barry to compromise the standards of European medical professionalism that she insisted upon. Dr Liesching (who was not a properly qualified medical man) took it for granted that his son, who had served five years after his apprenticeship as managing partner in his father's shop, would be allowed to open his own establishment. Barry, who was a stickler for standards, did not consider that the younger Liesching had the requisite qualifications. Her report on medical practice reveals something of her attitude to medicine as a vocation.

It was, she believed, vital to uphold the laws of the profession, since they were founded upon 'the most Honourable as well as useful' principles, and set up for the safety and welfare of the community at large. In medical practice, she pointed out, 'the lives of many must . . . be entrusted to the Discretion, Judgement and good faith of perhaps a single Individual'. Therefore no one could be permitted to become a candidate for examination or licensed to practise as physician, surgeon or apothecary without a qualification from a European university or college. Not only did her principles antagonize the local merchants, they also brought her sharply into conflict with the authorities.

Since it was impossible to acquire the correct qualifications in the Colony, the Supreme Medical Committee had in the past been content to turn a blind eye on the deficiencies of practitioners. Thus Dr Liesching senior was 'permitted rather than licensed' to practise as an apothecary and a surgeon. The privilege of practising without paper qualifications was jealously guarded but Barry was determined to uphold those professional standards she herself had struggled to acquire. She would not give in. In her opinion the state of medicine at the Cape was 'tolerably respectable' and 'allowing an unqualified person to practise would do untold harm since the Physician, Surgeon and the Patient are totally at the Mercy of the Chemist and druggist'.

All through the year the Lieschings, who were an influential family, bombarded Lord Charles both personally and in writing with memoranda pleading for an examination. The chemist's son complained that he was being discriminated against as a foreigner; he grumbled that Barry did not like him, that his wife and children were 'doomed to poverty and disgrace because it was Dr James Barry's pleasure'.

Lord Charles was under a great deal of pressure himself. He sent the application to the Chief Justice, who had already been lobbied by the Liesching family. The Chief Justice ruled that according to the law of the Cape a European diploma was not necessary for apothecaries, chemists, etc.; they merely needed certificates of apprenticeship and an examination in the Colony. 'Mr Liesching', wrote Sir John, 'had been employed in one of the first Apothecary shops in this town.'

Barry would have none of it. She assembled a board which included Dr Bailey, the founder of the Somerset Hospital, and two qualified apothecaries. These medical men found Mr Liesching ineligible for examination. And Barry was rash enough to declare publicly that Sir John Truter, the Chief Justice, 'could in no way be a judge or lay down the Law respecting the medical profession in any of its branches'. A gallant defence of medicine, but unwise; soon the whole legal establishment turned against her. The Fiscal, legal adviser to the Crown, felt that the authority of the Judiciary was at stake and firmly upheld the Chief Justice. In December the new Secretary to Government, Sir Richard Plasket, a civil servant of twenty-seven years' standing, with a considerable regard for his own importance, wrote to Barry telling her the Governor desired her to examine Mr Liesching. 'Dr Barry', noted Sir Richard, 'did not take the slightest notice.' Sir Richard wrote again and a fortnight later Barry answered that 'with becoming deference to the construction put by the legal advisers to the Government on the admission of medical men to practice' she herself felt that to examine Mr Liesching would be 'inconsistent with a sense of right in the conscientious discharge of my Professional duty'.

She suggested, tongue in cheek, a possible solution. Since the case was anomalous 'I humbly leave to His Excellency's consideration to dispense with an examination and grant to Mr Charles Liesching a licence to practise or otherwise as shall seem meet to His Excellency'. Barry's impudence infuriated the Government House officials. And only her privileged relationship with Lord Charles allowed it to go unpunished. Was she secretly enjoying this assertion of her independence? No doubt she wanted to make her own professional integrity absolutely plain – and provoke Lord Charles into the bargain.

The argument lasted over a year. Another Medical Board was appointed who were pleased to say 'yes' to Mr Liesching and pronounce him fully competent to start business as an independent apothecary. Mr Liesching was duly granted a licence, but in Sir Richard's view Dr Barry had forced the Government to act illegally. No person, according to law, was entitled to hold licence as physician or apothecary without the recommendation of the Colonial Medical Inspector.

Despite official letters flying back and forth and all the trouble that Barry was causing the Governor with her tiresome and repeated demands for reform, the curious bond between them held. Wherever Lord Charles Somerset appeared, Barry was sure to be near at hand. Their liaison had always been a subject for gossip. In a year of such simmering discontent it provoked more. One day, so the story went, Barry turned up at the Dutch Reformed Church for Sunday-morning service, and saw that the Governor's pew was empty. Without a moment's hesitation she turned on her heel and marched straight out again!

This gave the wits of the town a laugh – and a rhyme.

With courteous devotion inspired
Barry came to the temple of prayer
But quickly turned round and retired
When he found that HIS Lord was not there!

In quieter times the strange friendship between Barry and Lord Charles might have provoked no more than that kind of doggerel and some malicious laughter. But in the troubled atmosphere of the Cape their relationship inevitably provided ammunition for political attacks on the Government. Public discontent with the handling of the £50 000 voted by Parliament to be used for defraying the expense of the settlers combined with the inefficient defence of the frontier and dissatisfaction at the administration of civil affairs by the military to create an ugly mood.

Against the background of the Commission of Inquiry, which, by now, was well under way, the Colony's press used its newly acquired freedom to print harsh criticisms of the Cape Government. By May 1824 the administration was sufficiently alarmed by the attacks mounted in the new paper, the *South African Commercial Advertiser*, to take action. Two months earlier a notary called Edwards had been tried for libelling a Government officer and his references to the Governor as 'a Gambler, a Horse Jockey and a Cock Fighter, A Black Leg driven from Newmarket' were widely reported; in addition his remarks about 'little Barry' were heard by a packed courtroom.

Now Edwards was to be tried for libelling the Governor in his outbursts in court and the public were eagerly awaiting fresh disclosures. This alarmed the authorities. Determined to suppress the 'most contemptible marks of calumny and malice of the prisoner', the Fiscal, Mr Denyssen, took action. He descended on the newspaper offices and demanded to see proofs of the paper containing the report of the trial. From the publishers he extracted a promise that nothing 'scurrilous' should appear, and demanded 10 000 rix dollars as security. In the circumstances the publishers decided that it was their duty 'as British subjects to discontinue the publication'.

Two days later the *South African Journal*, a bi-monthly magazine, had also suffered a visit from the Fiscal and, as a result, that publication too had decided to close down: as the editors, Thomas Pringle and John Fairbairn, explained to the Fiscal, 'In consequence of your official communication . . . we think it inconsistent with our safety to continue publication.'

By now not only the British settlers, but the public at large were seething with indignation. On May 26th a memorandum with over 200 signatures was sent to the King 'praying' for a free press, 'the birthright of Englishmen and the firmest support and glory of their native country'.

Meanwhile criticism of the administration went underground. A series of malicious posters appeared mysteriously on the brick side of a house in the Herrengracht, the town's busiest street where Dr Barry lodged.

On June 1st, 1824, the settlers awoke to the news that a scurrilous placard had been pasted up near Dr Barry's house. By midday it had disappeared but two eyewitnesses swore that it had contained a 'foul slander' linking the names of Lord Charles Somerset and his personal physician. The news caused a sensation. The infamous placard, designed, so the Fiscal wrote, 'to wound the heart' of his Excellency the Governor, was immediately investigated at the Worshipful Court of Justice at the Cape.

Captain John Findlay, a Scotsman and master of the brig *Alacrity*, was the most important witness. He was in the habit of rising early, to look out for ships approaching port. His evidence is recorded as follows:

on Tuesday the 1st of June about 7 O'clock in the morning in coming on my stoep I saw a Libel fixed on the right side of the bridge . . . I went to the spot to learn the contents of it. I saw two persons unknown to me standing there, the one black of complexion and the other yellow . . . the yellow person, being a boy of about sixteen years of age, mentioned to me unasked that it was something about Lord Charles. I then examined that paper which I found to commence with the words 'a person' and to have been nearly of the contents ****

(At this point the exact wording of the report was censored!)

Another witness, Thomas Deane from Ireland, 'saw two slave boys with baskets on their heads and a person with a grey coat' at about sunrise. 'On looking at the post of the Bridge I heard them utter the words **** on which I dressed myself.'

The court hearing produced nothing more conclusive. The precise content of the placards seems to have eluded even the official records: the Dutch clerk, apparently, did not know how to spell the four letter word! One version mentioned 'Dr Barry's little wife'. The meaning was clear: Lord Charles and Dr Barry enjoyed an illicit relationship. Within hours Barry's name was bandied round the town.

Barry broke down and wept openly at Saunders (the confectioners) because of the affair, Mr Van der Sandt, a compositor in the Government Printing Office, said in evidence given during the court hearing. The incident brought into the open the rumours and sniggers about Barry and the Governor. Because people had speculated since her arrival at the Cape that Barry was a woman, the idea that she was Lord Charles's mistress must have been in many minds. One malicious person even suggested sending a copy of the 'foul libel' to Lady Charles Somerset. Those who accepted the peppery little doctor as a man must, on the other hand, have suspected a homosexual relationship. What the words 'Dr Barry's little wife' meant is as dead as the slang of the day, but that June the guesses, the hints and innuendoes were debated openly and with gusto under the guise of moral indignation. The 'heinous crime' remained a favourite topic. Coachmen and farm labourers sniggered about the placard over a bottle of wine at The Sign of the Sun. Officers whispered about it in the mess and the merchants and ladies talked endlessly in the gracious gardens of Government House.

Some people went so far as to suggest that the Governor himself had been responsible for the placard in order to win sympathy from the people and to gain the opportunity to blacken some dangerous enemies at the Cape, namely the dissident settlers who were causing him so much trouble. And, in fact, during the hunt for the villains the Fiscal had the homes of two troublesome settlers searched – the lawyer, Mr Edwards, who was by now in prison for libelling the Governor, and Mr Bishop Burnett, a farmer who had been declared bankrupt and ordered out of his home. Burnett, who was to play an increasingly damaging role in publicizing Lord Charles's 'vices', came nearer to the truth than he realized when he wrote that Barry 'is, has been and if rumour speaks true, will remain single'.

Lord Charles offered 5000 rix dollars reward for information and another 1000 rix dollars for the papers. In a proclamation he stated that 'Some ill-designed person . . . maliciously wrote and stuck up . . . a certain defamatory libel, tending to disgrace my character and honour and that of one of the officers of the Government.'

The merchants who had, of course, to demonstrate their loyalty to the Governor, offered to subscribe another 14000 rix dollars. But no one needed to pretend to a loyalty to Barry. She herself offered 1000 rix dollars reward for the discovery of the culprit. The reward finally stood at 21000 rix dollars (£1575). But the search, the court hearings, the financial inducement produced nothing.

News of the scurrilous placard – although not of its contents – had reached London. On the 21st of August 1824 the *Morning Chronicle* quoted a report from the *Cape Town Gazette*, the official Government paper, designed to show that the Governor's personal popularity was unaffected by the scandal. Soon after the placard appeared Lord Charles, the paper reported, had visited the theatre where an enthusiastic crowd greeted him: 'Proof if proof were necessary of the detestation excited by the vile calumnies of a concealed libeller.' The paper does not record whether Lord Charles's party was accompanied by his household physician. But for her the harm had been done. She had been openly mocked at the Cape. And within a year an even more shocking libel was to come to light.

Fortunately she was very busy. Earlier in the year an epidemic fever had broken out in the interior and a handful of families had died. As always, Barry responded to the emergency quickly and energetically. She called all the medical practitioners and apothecaries to her house in the Cape at ten o'clock one April morning, and outlined her plan of attack. Two large tablespoonfuls of turpentine, two of castor oil and one of water or peppermint water were to be taken; two hours later the patient was to be dosed with warm soup or tea. The medicine was to be repeated if it failed to work within twenty-four hours. The patient was also to be immersed for twenty minutes in a warm bath, with two or three bottles of Cape vinegar, and a towel moistened with cold vinegar was to be wrapped round the sufferer's head. Once back in bed, the patient was to be dosed with warm wine and water tinged with lemon juice. No wonder they labelled it her 'Wonderful Cape Punch'.

Above all, Barry believed in simple hygiene. The attendants were ordered to pay strict attention to personal cleanliness, to allow no visitors and to change linen daily: 'Want of cleanliness renders most diseases virulent, which by care would be of little consequence.' Her commonsense helped to contain the disease.

She began to assume even more responsibility. She had, by her own wish, become a medical inspector of the 'Tronk', the town prison, and in April of 1824 she visited it with Judge Kekewich (a friend of Lord Charles, and described by him as a 'mild, sensible, gentleman-like man'). They found a prisoner, one Jacob Elliot, in a dungeon with a fractured thigh and 'without clothes, without a bed or pillows or blankets, dirty in the extreme, without a single comfort and in short, exhibiting such a state of misery that if he had not been under the special protection of Providence he could not have survived'. The prisoner, with his warder looking on, told the official visitors that he had had no medicine and no proper diet except a bucket of water once a day and the common prison allowance. Until that morning he had been lying on the ground; only because official visitors were expected had a filthy stretcher been provided. 'I do here, my Lord, declare', Barry reported to the Governor, 'that I never witnessed any scene more truly appalling . . . Mr Kekewich went out in disgust.'

Barry felt bound to stay and find out if there were any more sick prisoners. She was shown a convict from Robben Island, Jan Krier, in a cell 'with one of his legs fractured and the other carefully surrounded with heavy chains'. She was appalled to discover that no beds or bedding were provided for the prisoners, that soup was served in tubs so that four or five prisoners had to slurp 'like pigs' to take their food. As for the women prisoners, they were dirty and wretched, and permitted no exercise in the fresh air at all – except for obligatory visits to church twice a week, Barry spoke personally to Lord Charles after she had visited the prisoners and said in her official report: 'I took the liberty of saying that if Your Excellency could afford the time to walk to the Tronk, you could satisfy yourself as to the facts and be convinced that I did not in the least exaggerate.'

She discussed the cases with the prison doctor and his son – her old enemies the Lieschings – who both assured her that *they* had asked to have Jacob Elliot transferred to hospital, and had even tried to provide him with clothes, bedding, and so on. 'They were very pleased that Your Excellency had been so good as to order the poor people into hospital and very anxious that you should see the official Reports which must now be lying on Mr Ryneveld's table.'

Barry seems to have accepted the Lieschings' assurance unquestioningly. Since Dr Liesching had recently advertised his refusal to continue to treat patients who could not afford to pay their bills (most medical men at the Cape prescribed free for needy patients) she was being a little naïve in taking his word. Mr Ryneveld was the Deputy Fiscal and, by accepting the Lieschings' explanation that they had requested the transfer, Barry was implicitly accusing Mr Ryneveld of negligence.

Mr Ryneveld got to hear of her remarks (for there were no secrets in the inner circle of Cape society) and he resented them. The Acting Colonial Secretary, Mr P. C. Brink, tried to warn her in a friendly way that she was making dangerous enemies, and even went so far as to show her a letter from Mr Ryneveld to prove his point.

She took umbrage. She thanked the Acting Colonial Secretary for allowing her to see Mr Ryneveld's letter with its complaint but added,

Dr James Barry begs to say that he is at a loss to understand its meaning; as every man in a Public situation must be aware that official duties neither might nor can become the subject of private 'altercations'. Upon this principle Dr James Barry considers it his bounden duty to disclaim anything like personalities in his official correspondence; but at the same time he must and will perform his public duties fearlessly and conscientiously and he again repeats that he does not, he cannot condescend ever to be personal. '*Honi soit qui mal y pense*' is the Englishman's motto.

No man in public office would have been as jealous of a

gentleman's honour. But Barry was a convert to the code of gentlemanly conduct, committed to uphold it even at an intellectual level. 'Good form' was not enough for her – she needed to believe in the innate chivalry of a gentleman in order to maintain her masquerade.

However, her passionate reports did prompt Lord Charles to ask her to visit and report on the prison and the Somerset Hospital officially. The Fiscal, too, was told that because of 'the wretched and appalling state' in which Dr Barry had found two prisoners, separate quarters must be provided for the sick in prison, and Dr Barry was to be afforded every facility for her visits. The Burgher Senate (in charge of the Somerset Hospital) received the same instructions.

In the meantime, Lord Charles Somerset himself was in trouble. Earl Bathurst at the Colonial Office was constantly intervening: asking for more details about expenditure at the Cape, complaining about extravagance, inquiring about judicial proceedings. The Commissioners of Inquiry, too, patiently investigated complaints that grew more vociferous almost daily. The Governor was personally charged with 'corruptly making a grant of land for a sum of money amounting to £750 under the colour and pretence of the sale of a horse'. The charge was never proved. The horse, a colt named Sorcerer, was said to be the finest ever seen in the Colony. Lord Charles, who had a genuine passion for horseflesh, had imported thirty-four thoroughbred English horses at considerable expense to himself on his return from England in 1821. Although in other ways the Governor might, with some justice, have been accused of exploiting his position, ironically his desire to improve bloodstock in the Cape was unquestionably sincere. And the Colony benefited from his initiative.

Under pressure Lord Charles became more autocratic. He banned the formation of a Literary Society at the Cape, and on December 20th *The Times* commented scathingly on his high-handed action. 'So much for colonial freedom under a Tory of the blood of a Somerset', it thundered. 'Was the Hottentot Grandee to be recalled?'

The disgruntled English settlers contributed to the unrest. The Fiscal, Mr Denyssen, was one of the Dutch officials who most resented their presence in the Colony. He was particularly disgruntled by Barry's report on the prison. His response was to set a trap for her: Aaron Smith was a drunken sailor who broke into the Fiscal's house one night, in a belligerent mood, and was sent to prison to cool off. Obligingly, the prison doctor, Dr Liesching, declared the man Smith 'deranged in his mind'. As Colonial Medical Inspector, Dr Barry was asked to recommend Smith's transfer to the lunatic asylum in August 1825. On the 25th August she examined the man and categorically refused to certify him mad. It is hard to believe that Plasket, the Fiscal and Dr Liesching, who had all smarted under Barry's tongue, did not foresee her reaction.

In her report she said:

Aaron Smith is perfectly sane in mind and by no means a subject for the Somerset Hospital . . . probably H.M. Fiscal's application for Aaron Smith's admission into that establishment has been in the spirit of 'pure charity' for the benevolent purpose of having the wounds inflicted upon this poor man by the Dienaars [constables] . . . professionally attended . . . [but] Dr Liesching [the prison doctor] said that within the last four days he considered him perfectly sane . . . and during the whole of confinement he did not think it necessary to give him a single dose of Physic or to make any alteration in his diet from the common prison allowance and only directed solitary confinement. I think it expedient to enter into this detail for the purpose of explaining that the absence of vinous and spiritous liquors was sufficient to restore Smith to his senses *such as they are.*

In that last sentence Barry shows herself to be unsentimental though compassionate where a drunken, maltreated prisoner was concerned. But she had allowed herself to snipe at the Fiscal, the man in charge of both prison and police force – and a dangerous enemy.

Acting on his own authority Sir Richard Plasket maliciously sent a copy of the report, intended for the Governor, to the Fiscal, on the pretext that the latter should look into this 'apparently disgraceful business'.

To her surprise, eighteen days after her first visit to the prison Dr Barry was again ordered to examine and certify the wretched Smith, this time described as 'raving mad'. Barry had believed that the prisoner was to be discharged the day after her *first* visit. If that had been done, she wrote in her official report, Smith could not have been in his present melancholy state. On her second visit Barry decided that it was Smith's presence in the Tronk which was in itself 'sufficient to induce madness in any person whose mind has ever before been affected'. She considered him ill and weak, with his mind partially deranged, a case for 'professional treatment in hospital although not a lunatic asylum' unless he deteriorated.

In this letter Barry again shows herself to be years ahead of her time – indeed, she would be regarded as enlightened even today. She was suggesting that madness should be treated in hospital, not in an asylum. She also believed that the environment could induce insanity.

The Colonial civil servants who read her reports could not begin to understand her approach. They were not concerned with the niceties of medicine. They were not even concerned with the fate of Aaron Smith. It was Dr Barry, with her arrogance, her intemperate language, and above all her thinly disguised attacks on dignataries and institutions, that upset them.

The day that Barry wrote her second report on the prisoner she was summoned to appear before the local Court of Justice to be examined about her previous statement to the Governor. She was furious. According to Plasket, Dr Barry 'tore up the summons and threw it in the messenger's face'. She was summoned again and duly appeared in Court but refused to take the oath, answer questions or say one word in her capacity as Colonial Medical Inspector. If her reports to the Governor were to be 'shackled' then it would prevent public officers from bringing to light those very abuses that ought to be brought to His Excellency's notice, she believed. Mr Denyssen, the Fiscal, grew purple with rage at her silence. He ruled that Dr Barry should be put in prison for a month if she persisted in her objections. At that moment a messenger appeared, with a note for Dr Barry, requiring her immediate attendance on the 'Lady of Colonel Somerset' (Lord Charles's daughter-in-law) who was indisposed. It could hardly have been a coincidence.

At noon the next day the Court reassembled. Barry appeared punctually, but again she refused to speak. She was sentenced to civil imprisonment. At once she penned a note to Lord Charles. 'I am advised to throw myself upon your Lordship to protect the Liberty of a Public Officer who has not transgressed a law . . . the only charge against whom is that of having conscientiously discharged a public duty, imposed by your Excellency.'

Barry took the letter herself to the Governor, supported by Judge Kekewich and Mr Bigge, one of the Commissioners of Inquiry. The Governor sent for the Fiscal and after an hour's conference he suspended the sentence.

The Fiscal, of course, denied any brutality to the prisoners, and Lord Charles was obviously embarrassed and annoyed by the whole affair. Once again Dr Barry was brought into the public eye under his protection – and only three months after the placard affair. Sir Richard Plasket told the Commissioners of Inquiry that he 'spoke strongly to the Governor' about her several times. (He was, more and more, assuming authority.) The result was a letter of reproof penned by Sir Richard in the Governor's name.

His Excellency desires me to say that whatever appearance there may have been of the ill-treatment of Aaron Smith, or of the probability of such ill-treatment [*Barry had, in fact, asked several of the other prisoners about it*] . . . *His Excellency cannot refrain from remarking on the very great impropriety of your indulging yourself in reflections on the character of His Majesty's Fiscal.*

Barry was incapable of accepting a curb on her professional freedom even from Lord Charles. She consulted Colonel Bell, an army friend, about her position as a British officer threatened with civil imprisonment. He considered she had suffered an injustice and advised her to tell the two Commissioners of Inquiry about it. (They were both her patients, recommended to her by Lord Charles.)

She went straight to Sir Richard Plasket's office to ask for copies of documents about the trial. On the way she met Colonel Bird (the Governor's ex-secretary, now out of favour). 'I am astonished to see you at liberty', he called from his dogcart, 'I was on my way to the Tronk to leave my card.' Barry nearly exploded.

She had difficulty in getting in to see Sir Richard. And when she did he seems to have tried to placate her. She pointed out that it was he who had caused the trouble by passing her private report to the Governor on to the Fiscal. She intended, she told him, to place the documents of the case before the Commissioners.

'If you do, you shall be dismissed from your situation and I shall recommend it', answered the Governor's Secretary. 'Indeed, Sir,' returned Barry, 'now you have threatened, I will do so, not as a matter of complaint, but for their opinion and investigation as well as for my own edification.'

Inevitably, the interview turned into a slanging match. Barry reminded the Colonial Secretary that she was the member of a board *ordered* to inquire into the state of the prisons; Sir Richard rebuked her for her 'improper' language. But Barry had the last word. She told the pusillanimous civil servant that if she had had her sword on when 'Mr Fiscal proposed sending me to the Tronk, I should most certainly have cut off both his Ears, his Jews' Ears off to make him look smart'.

It was an impossible situation. Sir Richard Plasket was concerned 'to uphold the Government and to support its dignity and authority'. Barry's 'bullying and brow-beating the local authorities' could only undermine it. He could not concern himself with the plight of the prisoners or the conditions of the sick: he was aloof, remote from such people. But for Barry the question of the prisoners was a question of her duty. Had she not reported on the bruises and wounds on Aaron Smith, she would not have felt herself fit to hold her high office. The two simply did not understand each other.

Meanwhile, Lord Charles's own position was deteriorating rapidly. Sir Richard Plasket had recently written home to R. Wilmot Horton, the Under Secretary of State for the Colonies, observing that 'almost every single Department under this Government is in a state of total incompetence'. Just at the time that Barry was facing civil imprisonment, the Government at the Cape had received news of the debates in the House of Commons 'on the conduct of Lord Charles Somerset'. The ship *Caesar* brought the newspapers 'which pointed out that leave of absence had been granted to Lord Charles' to go home and face the charges against him in person. Plasket noted that Lord Charles seemed 'very anxious'.

Since the debate had, of course, revived the placard affair and attacked Lord Charles's 'honor and character', any further public protection of Dr Barry must have seemed too dangerous. On June 16th, 1825 an even more scandalous version of the libel had actually been repeated in the House of Commons. It accused Lord Charles of committing 'an unspeakable atrocity with his reputed son, the household physician'.

In short Dr Barry was an embarrassment. The Government at the Cape – and most particularly the Secretary to the Governor – wanted to drop her. 'His Excellency the Governor was impressed', wrote Plasket, 'with the impropriety of any one individual being entrusted with the sole management and control of the Colonial Medical Department'.

Impropriety was the key word. In Plasket's view Barry held too much personal influence. The solution was to be a Medical Board which would take over the wide-ranging responsibilities of the Colonial Medical Inspector. Since Barry was such a junior officer she could not possibly become President. Instead Dr Arthur, Principal Military Medical Officer (who had proved tractable to the Governor's wishes in the Liesching affair), was to head the Board which would administer the functions previously performed by Barry alone. Through the gossips of the Cape, she learned that she was to be offered no more than a seat on it. 'We intend giving you a seat on *our* Committee . . .' Sir Richard himself told her haughtily.

Her enemies were shrewd. They realized that since she had run the Colonial Medical Department, had in fact *been* the Colonial Medical Department she would never accept a subordinate position.

Through an expression, a turn of phrase in her report on the prison, which was in her view necessary for the public good, she was to be outlawed from civil duties. The injustice of it prompted her to write endless letters of protest.

To clarify her position, she asked to be allowed to attend a meeting of the Colony's Supreme Council on the 28th of October, when the matter of the Colonial Medical Department was to be debated. Her request was refused. At the meeting, no inquiry into the state of the Medical Department was made and no inspection either of medicines, or of drugs, or of practice of medicine, was even discussed. It was clear that Dr Barry, not the Department, was on trial.

The outcome was a foregone conclusion. The office of the Colonial Medical Inspector was to be abolished and a Supreme Medical Committee appointed in its stead.

Actually Barry had anticipated the decision and had already written her resignation:

> I lose no time in requesting to intimate to your Lordship that it will be impossible for me to reconcile to my feelings the acceptance of any subordinate place in the proposed Establishment. In this event, I beg respectfully to tender my resignation of the Civil Situations that I hold and I request to be honoured with an early communication of your Lordship's final intentions, before they are made Public in order that I may decide on the arrangements that will become necessary under such an alternative.

That 'the favourite of the family', the inseparable companion of Lord Charles, was driven to write in terms like these, suggests just how hurt she was, both personally and professionally. She did not object to a board being formed – she had already said so. But it was impossible for anyone, let alone the proud and impetuous Dr Barry, to serve as a junior in a department she had once ruled single-handed.

The next day Lord Charles wrote back, repeating the complaints about her 'very improper language' which had so greatly embarrassed the authorities, and 'the imputations you unsparingly and unreservedly cast upon Officers of this Government'. The Governor told her that his secretary, Sir Richard Plasket, had felt it his duty to recommend the restoring of the Medical Committee. Lord Charles added:

> I observed that it would be certainly beneficial and that the only obstacle was my apprehension that it *might hurt your feelings* as Dr Arthur must be a Member, and as you were a Military Officer, of course, he must take place of you . . . As Sir Richard conceives from his conversation with you yesterday that you impute to him personal motives of hostility towards you which I can venture to assert he has not . . . I shall at his request submit the whole of the correspondence for the consideration of the Council.

Was it an apology? That the Governor should refer to Barry's 'feelings' in an official document after her 'improper behaviour' must surely reflect his own unease. The fact was that the Council and Government could hardly be more embarrassed – 'attacked from every side and quarter' as Lord Charles himself wrote in a letter home. One cannot escape the impression that Lord Charles was a frightened man.

If Barry was removed from high office, no doubt both Sir Richard and Lord Charles fervently hoped that they would hear no more of her. Of course they did.

The Commissioners of Inquiry took up Barry's case. At her suggestion, they had seen for themselves the state of the prison and the hospital. As far as they were concerned, the most serious aspect of the affair was that if civil servants were warned off giving evidence, then the Commission could not do its work and the true state of affairs in the Colony could not be uncovered and improved. As it was, rumour whispered that spies were loitering in the lobbies of Government House, close by the Commissioners' office, to check who went in and to find out their business. The Commissioners had already noticed a certain 'reluctance' in civil servants to talk freely about official matters.

Concerned, the Commissioners wrote endless letters to Sir Richard about the affair. Sir Richard, in his turn, wrote back listing his reasons for advising Dr Barry's dismissal. He brought up the Liesching controversy, and singled out what he described as Barry's most impertinent letter refusing to recognize the Chief Justice's right 'to be a Judge or lay down the Law respecting the Medical Profession'.

He argued that Barry herself had recommended the appointment of a board to settle that affair. He referred to the merchants' memorandum against her and the recent scandal of the case of Aaron Smith.

Sir Richard protested that he had neither time nor memory to recall Barry's 'numerous improprieties', but permitted himself to allude to three. Barry's first offence had been to 'set up a kind of Horse Whistle' during the interview at Government House about her prison sentence, while the Governor Lord Charles was explaining to Judge Kekewich how the Fiscal had defended his conduct in summoning Barry. Her 'Horse Whistle' is in fact solemnly noted in the Records of the Cape Colony.

The second impropriety occurred at 'a meeting of the Bachelors' to arrange a ball for Lady Charles Somerset. On that occasion, apparently, Dr Barry had attacked the Secretary to the Commission of Inquiry and alluded to the long stay of the commissioners in the Colony.

Thirdly, Sir Richard said that he had met Barry after the interview in his office and she had apologized for the violence of her temper. Sir Richard said:

I told him I thought nothing of it. I merely wanted him to listen to reason. I begged of Dr Barry to write to Government if he still refused a seat on the Medical Board to ask leave to be excused, to submit to the new arrangement in the Medical Department and suggest that his services might give him a claim on Government for something else.

Barry would not be appeased. Sir Richard, exasperated, told her that he would have nothing more to do with the case individually. The subject would come up before Council. 'Before Council – much good I shall get from that', she retorted. 'What can I expect from Sir John Truter? [The Chief Justice whom Barry had antagonized over the Liesching affair.] As to Mr Stoll he is a connection of Dr Liesching.' Too late Barry was realizing that she had made too many dangerous enemies in Cape society.

Meanwhile Sir Richard Plasket was intriguing against her. In December 1825 he complained to his friend Horton at the Colonial Office of the 'personal influence which Dr Barry exercises' over the Commissioners of Inquiry. He also begged that Horton would refer to Sir James McGrigor (Director of the Army Medical Department) for information about Dr Barry's conduct in his military professional character 'which, I understand, has been frequently complained of, by His Superior Officers'.

Sir Richard reserved his most damning comment to the last. 'I have only one thing to say in Dr Barry's favor . . . that he has been spoiled by Lord Charles originally, and by the Commissioners of Enquiry latterly who have allowed him to do and say just what he pleased.' Sir Richard does not attempt to explain the reason for Barry's 'personal influence' with the Commissioners. Nor for the 'spoiling'.

For her part, Barry, sent, via the Commissioners, a review of her service in office as Colonial Medical Inspector, and closed with a flourish.

Thus, in the midst of public and important duties, scarcely yet completed I was disgracefully virtually dismissed from my Office. And I must here repeat, to the utter ruin of my professional character and prospects in Life. As to the temporary inconvenience of pecuniary matters, I have not, I do not give them a thought. I had, indeed, flattered myself that I was bartering my time, my health and my talents (such as they are) to the Public Benefit, for honest fame, not sacrificing them to infamy.

It did not help. She lost her post as Colonial Medical Inspector, her official standing as Lord Charles's physician and most of her salary. Her pay in 1826 as Assistant Staff Surgeon was just 7s. 6d. a day.

It was a poor reward for two and a half years' service. She had, however, improved conditions in the prison and hospital and laid the foundations for reform. Perhaps her most important contribution was to introduce new standards of hygiene and a new attitude to public health in the Colony. One of her last acts as Colonial Medical Inspector had been to replace the capital's open sewers by sealed iron pipes.

As for Lord Charles, he was a man at bay. In March of 1826, advised by Sir Richard Plasket and by Lord Bathurst, he finally acknowledged the broad hints thrown out by Parliament and agreed to come home and face his accusers.

At eleven-fifteen on the morning of 5th March, His Excellency Lord Charles Somerset, Governor of the Cape of Good Hope and Commander in Chief of the Forces, embarked on the *Atlas* China ship. As a local newspaper reported:

From early in the morning, Government House was crowded with visitors who came to take their leave. A few minutes after eleven, His Excellency with his staff left Government House on horseback, escorted by Lt. General Bourke, and the Commissioners of Enquiry. Lady Charles travelled in her carriage with Miss Somerset, Lady C. Bell, Lady M. Fitzroy, and others. Soldiers in red coats lined the street from Government House to the Parade. When His Excellency entered the Government barge, he was accompanied by Lady Charles and Miss Somerset . . . and Dr Barry.

Loyalty was one of Barry's most enduring qualities. Despite public odium and private disappointment, she demonstrated her allegiance to the Governor on his departure. It is somehow pleasing to report that her arch enemy, the Governor's secretary, who had so much resented Barry's intimate friendship with Lord Charles, followed in the next boat.

All the ships in the bay were richly decorated with colours and as the barge passed the tars gave three hearty cheers. On the *Helicon* a salute of thirteen guns was fired. The visitors lingered on board as long as it was possible and did not leave the ship till the Captain announced that she was under weigh . . .

For nearly ten years Barry had been the Governor's protégée, the family favourite. Now she was, so it seemed, relegated to a junior officer's post, destined to live in oblivion.

6

'To rescue my good name . . .'

Despite her fears of professional ruin, seven months after she was stripped of civilian office Dr Barry scored her most brilliant success as a surgeon.

A wealthy snuff merchant in Cape Town, Thomas Munnik, sent an urgent message to Barry to come to his wife who was desperately ill in labour. Barry rushed to the scene, examined Mrs Munnik and made a lightning decision: on July 25th, 1826, on the kitchen table of the Munnik home, she operated, making an incision into the abdomen. She delivered the baby, a healthy boy, by Caesarian section; then in a matter of minutes she sewed up Mrs Munnik's wound and saved her life.

In those days, before anaesthetics or antiseptics, the dangers of infection or of fatal post-operative shock were daunting. Life depended on the surgeon's skill and, above all, speed. To save both mother and child was nothing short of a miracle. Barry's Edinburgh training must have prompted her decision to operate – Alexander Hamilton, the father of her own professor of midwifery, had been one of the first medical men of the eighteenth century to admit that a Caesarian was justified in certain cases. As a student she had had the operation described but had never seen it performed. Her success brought her widespread acclaim in the Cape Colony, and the Munnik family, who were close friends of Dr Barry, remained permanently grateful to her. She refused to accept a fee for her services, but at her own request the baby was named after her, and she was invited to become the godfather. At the baptism held in the Lutheran Church in Cape Town, Assistant Surgeon James Barry, in full-dress uniform, held the baby in her arms. For over 100 years the custom of naming the firstborn Munnik sons after James Barry has continued. (The present James Barry Munnik is himself a doctor, a psychiatrist in South Africa.)

Although at the time the family did not suspect her sex, they did want a portrait of her as a keepsake. She was understandably reluctant, so her likeness was taken by stealth and a portrait from the sketch painted on ivory. The family hold old newspaper cuttings, the portrait, a letter and a wealth of stories about Dr Barry. Today they are convinced that she was a woman.

In 1826 she was a woman disappointed. Although she believed, until it was impossible to believe it any longer, that 'Lord Charles Somerset's sense of justice would induce him to see me righted', as she put it, her faith in him was never justified. During 1826 she heard from friends in England that false tales had been told about her to Lord Bathurst at the Colonial Office (she was said to be a supporter of the Governor's enemy, Colonel Bird). To her, it must have seemed like government by gossip.

She wrote to Earl Bathurst complaining that to her 'utter astonishment I have been much misrepresented to your Lordship'. She had, she said, told her friend Sir Jahleel Brenton, who was now living in London, the whole story. 'Sir Jahleel is authorised by me to communicate the same personally to your Lordship if necessary', she added, with a due sense of her own importance. Sir Jahleel, a fervent Christian and commander of the Royal Yacht, was an unimpeachable source.

Her silence until that time and her present 'backwardness' arose she wrote, 'from my sincere and ardent wish to do nothing that could in any way injure Lord Charles Somerset; but solely to rescue my good name from Dishonor'.

Her letter crossed with one from Downing Street informing her that Earl Bathurst 'saw no reason to doubt the arrangement' which abolished her post as Colonial Medical Inspector and transferred the duties to a Medical Board.

She persisted. In a letter sent by return to this 'death blow to my hopes', she explained that it was not the abolition of the office that she objected to, but the 'injurious and disgraceful manner in which it was done'. Her job removed, her professional reputation defamed and her peace of mind destroyed . . . 'It is perhaps here needless for me to enforce how dear, how very dear to me my good name is', she added.

In fact the long, careful report of the Commissioners of Inquiry on the 'Case of Dr Barry' had by then already reached Downing Street. The report certainly vindicated her good name. Although the Commissioners found that Dr Barry had written in tones of 'unbecoming warmth'; that she should not have been so ready (in the affair of the drunken sailor, Aaron Smith) to impute to a constable consequences partly due to the man's own conduct, habits and conditions; they had the grace to add 'we are well aware that the conduct of the constable would justify [Barry's] epithets'.

They considered that Dr Barry should have been allowed to explain herself to the Governor in Council; that the Council should have considered 'whether the want of temper and discretion with which he was charged was not in some measure palliated and counterbalanced by his integrity and zeal . . . in bringing about reform of abuses'.

In fact they felt that Dr Barry should have been left in charge, with a board of leading doctors acting as referees to give sanction to her actions. But it was all too late. The post was abolished. The Supreme Medical Committee was in command.

That the Commissioners of Inquiry noted that, until the affair of Aaron Smith, Dr Barry's official business with the Chief Secretary and the Deputy Colonial Secretary had been conducted in a very friendly manner; and that her 'professional talents and reputation were universally acknowledged and by no person more emphatically than Lord Charles Somerset and his family' only underlined the irony of the situation. She was the best-known, best-respected, most-sought-after doctor in the Colony – and she was disgraced.

But despite her belief that 'military promotion may continue to be obstructed, if not annihilated', despite Sir Richard Plasket's malicious attempts to blacken her name at the Army Medical Department, she did gain promotion. On the 27th November 1827 Dr James Barry was gazetted Staff Surgeon.

For almost a year little was heard of her at the Cape. She was appointed to Mauritius but seems to have lingered, unwilling to leave the Colony with all its associations. On the 19th of September a permit for Dr Barry's servant, Dantzen, to leave for Mauritius was granted. The night before, in Cape Town, she held an official farewell party.

A local reporter described it:

The friends of Dr Barry with a view of marking their high opinion of his merits and of their regret at his departure to Mauritius on promotion, invited him to a dinner at George's Hotel on Monday last. The evening passed harmoniously, the dinner and wines were excellent. Health and prosperity to Dr Barry was drunk and the impression excited on Dr Barry was evident.

She apparently acknowledged the good wishes of the company 'with great taste and feeling'.

She had been twelve years at the Cape. She had fought one duel with pistols and several with the local administration. She had been praised as a 'prodigy' and mocked as mischievous and absurd. She had the highest reputation as a doctor and yet was described as a 'browbeating bully'. She had come out as an impressionable young girl of seventeen, and left a woman of twenty-nine, with considerable experience of power and political duplicity. But despite the storm of abuse that she aroused, and with a prison sentence over her head, even her most bitter enemies did not, dared not, attack her professional talent and integrity. She left the Colony as an officer and gentleman. Many years were to elapse before she was recognized as Cape Town's first social reformer.

On the 9th October, 1828 she landed on Mauritius. Mauritius, a small island in the Indian Ocean, was a much less attractive station. 'The streets were narrow and ill-disposed, the houses low, dark and dirty and inconvenient', wrote a traveller in 1829. When hurricanes came 'the houses rocked like cradles', the atmosphere, unlike the Cape, was unhealthy. The weather was often terribly hot and sultry but with a strong breeze.

Colonial life in Mauritius was even more riddled with gossip, protocol, and all the pettiness of a small community turned in on itself. Ladies struggled into full evening dress for Government House levées; tiffin was a ritual. The island boasted a beefsteak club and a ball was held somewhere or other every night. But the company to be found at these social functions was predictably familiar. After the excitement and vigour of life at Government House where she had frequently dined with visitors on the sea route to India, Mauritius must have seemed intolerably provincial to Barry. Her disgruntlement at her demotion was aggravated by a daily routine which offered her little stimulus.

Dr Barry, with her talent for trouble, was soon embroiled with the Governor. Two months after she arrived, the senior Civil and Military Medical Officer on the island, Dr McMullen, left for home due to ill-health. Sir Charles Colville, the Governor, proposed appointing Dr Shanks, Assistant Surgeon, of the 82nd Regiment – *junior* to Barry – in his place. He wrote home explaining his decision.

Among other applicants for the situation has been Doctor Barry, who within these two months, joined this force as Staff Surgeon and who as such will succeed to Dr McMullen as Head of the Military branch, but I have felt myself called upon to tell him that from his non-acquaintance with the French language, the climate of the Island, its habits and usages, I do not think him at present qualified for it.

The post needed, Sir Charles explained, 'much of local information and habits of acting with the functionaries and society of the island'. Dr Shanks had lived on Mauritius for eleven years and was a 'well-known, respected and consulted' doctor.

A postscript to the letter reveals a protest from Barry. 'Since writing the above I have learnt from Doctor Barry that I was in error respecting his ignorance of the French language.' Barry, it appears, *had* asked for an interpreter, on a visit to a patient, and someone had seen to it that the Governor had heard about it. But she had needed the interpreter for a Creole patient.

However, the Governor added, rather petulantly, this did not alter his preference for Dr Shanks.

Were it likely that a better knowledge of Dr Barry would have led to a different decision, he has only to thank himself for what he may have lost – for his absence at the Cape of Good Hope was of such duration after his appointment here, as to make it generally believed that he had no intention of taking it up.

Pique shows in that letter – pique towards Barry. But perhaps there is more to it than that. The Commissioners of Inquiry from the Cape, Barry's old friends Major Colebrooke and Mr Bigge, were on Mauritius at the time. Although they supported Barry, the story of the rumpus she had created at the Cape had surely reached the island. Her friendship with the two men who were investigating conditions under his authority was not likely to endear her to the Governor.

Another curious fact emerges from Sir Charles's letter. He assumes that Barry did not know the island. She herself writes in an official War Office record of her service that she was at Mauritius 'during the Cholera'. The outbreak was from November 1819 to January 1820, the very time that Lord Charles Somerset was away in England. Why did she not explain to Sir Charles Colville that she had spent some time on the island? Was it because she was trying to hide something – the birth of her baby, perhaps?

In the spring of 1829 she clashed again with authority. In February Mrs Fenton, the pregnant wife of an Indian Army officer bound for England on leave, stopped off at Mauritius to have her baby. The night Mrs Fenton's labour started her own doctor, Dr Shanks (the man who had taken precedence over Barry), was out visiting another patient. Mrs Fenton's nurse rushed over to the Regimental Mess and persuaded a young officer, Assistant Surgeon Dr Robinson, to come out to her patient. The Staff Surgeon was also called in and at four in the morning a baby girl, Flora, was delivered, safe and healthy.

According to Mrs Fenton, who kept a journal during her stay on the island, Dr Barry objected to the calling in of army doctors as 'highly irregular' and brought charges against Dr Robinson and the Staff Surgeon, Dr Hart. She disliked the practice of hospital doctors attending private patients and thus implicitly neglecting their hospital duties. Barry abided by her own high standards and expected others to do the same. At the

Cape, as Colonial Medical Inspector she had voluntarily taken on the visiting of the prison and the hospital, so she naturally disapproved of officers who accepted lucrative private work. It was a matter of principle and, like most of Barry's ideas, so far ahead of its time as to appear absurd or malicious. Barry was genuinely indignant, but as a junior officer she was exceeding her authority by interfering.

In her diary Mrs Fenton records that:

A Court of Inquiry was ordered to investigate the doctors. In the course of it, my own poor nurse, frightened out of her natural life in being sent for to prove that Mr Robinson [the junior officer involved] had left the hospital and was undressed and reading in his room when she went to beg his immediate attendance on me.

The Governor soon swept aside Barry's charges. 'Sir Charles Colville', says Mrs Fenton 'set the matter at rest by a general order fully acquitting the doctors.' The Governor insisted that Mrs Fenton 'being the wife of an old and meritorious officer had a right to the attendance of a regimental surgeon – especially in the absence of her husband'.

The incident could only have increased the Governor's initial dislike of Barry and Mrs Fenton even mentioned that 'there was some notice of removal to Dr Barry, the particulars of which I forget'.

At Mauritius, as at the Cape, there was someone who suspected her sex. Even before the arrival on the island, Mrs Fenton had enjoyed some unforgettable gossip about Barry. She confided to her journal that 'when visiting the sickroom of a friend in India she had chattered to the nurse in attendance who told a strange story about Dr Barry in Cape Town'. The nurse insisted that she had been driven out of the Cape by the little doctor, 'over whom there hung some extraordinary mystery'. The woman had been highly thought of and often attended on Dr Barry's cases, until one extraordinary night when she thought a patient she was tending urgently needed the doctor's care. Dr Barry was staying in the house of the sick lady, and when he did not appear immediately,

the nurse went herself and made an unceremonious entrance into the room. Thereon he flew into a violent passion. She declares and steadily maintains that Dr Barry was and is a woman. From this time he displayed the most implacable dislike to her, even to making it a condition not to attend in any family where she was employed.

Could Mrs Fenton have kept this extraordinary tale to herself? Or did it circulate around the island, so that within a few months of arrival Barry was, once again, an intriguing topic of conversation? Her journal was not published until 1901, long after Barry was dead and the scandal of her sex made public. Certainly the rumours of the story could not have reached Barry since she and Mrs Fenton remained friends despite the inquiry that followed Barry's complaints about the delivery of her baby.

In June 1829 Mrs Fenton noted in her diary that she had 'just put Flora in her basket, and set off on a pedestrian tour through this island with Dr Barry'. According to Mrs Fenton, Dr Barry was 'on the wing' like herself, so a tour of the island together seemed 'both agreeable and natural'. Unfortunately Mrs Fenton did not have any more to say about the mysterious Dr Barry or their trip together and she left the island soon afterwards.

So did Barry. On 27th August, barely ten months after she arrived on Mauritius, she sailed for England. She came home apparently without leave, and the tattle of the town suggests that she flouted her conduct at the authorities. *All the Year Round*, a magazine edited by Charles Dickens, wrote in 1867 (two years after Barry's death) the popular version of her meeting with her superiors after she had taken French leave.

'Sir', said Sir James McGrigor, the head of the Army Medical Department, 'I do not understand your reporting yourself in this fashion. You admit you have returned without leave of absence. May I ask you how this is?' 'Well', said James, coolly running his long white fingers through his crisp sandy curls, 'I have come home to have my hair cut!' Another explanation put forward for Barry leaving Mauritius so abruptly was that the Senior Medical Officer had read her a report about to be sent to the Horse Guards which described her as 'somewhat unfortunate in manner, lacking in tact and impatient of control'. Fair comment!

Barry herself gave her own explanation in an official memorandum at the close of her army career. 'I served (in the Mauritius) about eighteen months and was recalled *in consequence of the serious illness of Lord Charles Somerset.'*

If she was recalled, then no official letters about the incident survive. One tantalizing entry, however, exists in the Colonial Office papers, and simply notes a letter received from Dr Barry with the pencilled entry 'missing' beside it.

Since Lord Charles Somerset's brother Fitzroy, who had served in the Peninsular War with Wellington, was now Military Secretary at the Horse Guards, it seems plausible to suppose that Barry's return to England was the result of discreet pressure from above. Once more Lord Charles was seriously ill; he had unbounded faith in her skill as a doctor; whom else would he send for? She answered the call without hesitation. From everything we know about her, it is clear that she would put her personal feelings aside in the sickroom. Despite her disappointment over his behaviour towards her at the Cape, she never said a bitter word against Charles Somerset. Her actions speak of an unshakeable affection. Within two months of her arrival she had nursed the ex-Governor back to health.

By February 1830, Lord Charles was fit enough to be gazetted Colonel of the 33rd Regiment of Foot. However, Dr Barry did not return to Mauritius. She was, in fact, already overdue for her next posting – to Jamaica. A letter received by Sir James McGrigor reveals that approval had been given for Dr James Barry to leave for Jamaica on January 20th, 1830. But pencilled across it was a note 'bring down on September 1', amended later to 'bring down about September 25'.

Someone was delaying Barry's departure. Was it Fitzroy Somerset? Perhaps she was not quite certain about Lord Charles's recovery. Perhaps Lord Charles, always a hypochondriac, was loath to let his doctor go. They were still together on December 28th, over a year after Barry left Mauritius. On that day, Lord Charles drew up a will and 'James Barry, Surgeon to the Forces' was one of the witnesses to it.

In February 1831 Lord Charles went to fashionable Brighton for the weekend. On Sunday the 19th he was out riding. On the following day, 20th February, he died of a seizure. Strangely enough, this autocratic high Tory, who had so much enjoyed the pageantry of office, had asked to be buried 'with the least possible expense and on no account be attended with any parade'.

The *Brighton Gazette* reported that:

> the remains of Lord Charles were removed from the Bedford Hotel to the burial grounds attached to St Andrew's Chapel and deposited in a vault, being the first corpse interred there . . . The hearse was followed by three coaches and the mourners included his sons, brothers, with *the medical attendant* . . .

7

A Smell of Freedom

When Dr Barry arrived in Jamaica in June 1831 a smell of freedom was in the air. For over twenty years Parliament had been trying to persuade the planters to free the slaves on the sugar plantations. Now the slave-owners were threatened with financial sanctions in an attempt to force their acquiescence. The big estates were mostly owned by absentee landlords, but their managers lived a lordly life, with their great houses and fragrant gardens, their body slaves for every member of their family and their coloured mistresses. They were furious at Parliament's 'tyrannical' attitude and considered the threat of sanctions 'subversive to the sacredness of property'.

The slaves, of course, had heard the table talk of freedom while serving their masters; sometimes 'walking buckras' – discharged sailors or bookkeepers, who would travel the island, reading to the slaves in return for food, rum and lodging – brought the news to them. No doubt they did not fully understand the political background, but they were convinced that the King, William IV, wanted to set them free.

Perhaps it was fortunate for her professional career that Dr Barry had no official responsibility for the civilians on the island. Otherwise, with her reputation for freeing one slave and her outspoken sympathy for others, she would almost certainly have landed in trouble.

As it was, she was too busy caring for the health of the troops in an outpost which most of them regarded as a vast graveyard. Apart from Sierra Leone, the station had the worst health record in the Empire. One in nine of the British soldiers stationed there died every year between 1816 and 1836. (By contrast, the Cape Colony had a mortality rate of one in eighty-seven, the lowest in the Army at the time.)

In Jamaica, Barry's efforts to impose a régime of cleanliness and order, and thus improve the health of the troops in the eight military hospitals under her care, met with failure. The scorching sun and the wretched conditions in which the troops lived and died needed more drastic remedies than she could command. The soldiers were not kitted out for tropical service and took no precautions against sunstroke. The real killer, however, was the structure and the siting of the barracks; the soldiers' quarters were built on low, marshy ground, swarming with mosquitoes which carried the terrible yellow fever, or 'Yellow Jack', into dark barracks, stifling when doors were closed and shutters fastened on the wooden windows, and draughty when the trade winds blew. When the rains came, driving in great sheets across the island, damp seeped in and dripped all night on to the men, who huddled, shivering and sweating, on their hammocks. Unlike the officers, who had balconies built round their quarters, the men's barracks had balconies on one side only. Hygiene was primitive: the same wooden tubs served the troops as urinals and wash-bowls.

For their service, which could last as long as ten years if they survived, they were paid the princely sum of a shilling a day: of that 3s. 6d. was deducted for messing and 1s. 10½d. for washing and 'maintenance of necessaries'. They were lucky to have three-pence in their hands to spend. During the hot months, when the air was oppressively still, the men were confined to barracks by the sun from nine in the morning until four in the afternoon. All day long they had nothing to do except scratch at the mosquito bites and wait for the second of their two meals a day – salt beef and biscuits.

When they struggled out of doors in the afternoon, dazed by the heat, they naturally went in search of the one comfort that the island offered in abundance – rum. For a penny-halfpenny they could buy a pint of it – more than enough to guarantee oblivion. To quench their thirst, aggravated by the heat and their salt diet, they diluted the rum with water, a dangerous combination in that climate. (Even if they had wanted it, they could not have afforded the price of milk.) After sundown they became noisy and destructive – and that was followed by the lash; flogging was a daily and dreaded routine.

There was little else than drink to divert them on the island. No organized sport was provided and no facilities for recreation. Two out of three of the soldiers were illiterate, and even those who could read were restricted by the candle ration (two tallow dips to every twelve men). Very few soldiers had their wives with them. The Army permitted six wives to every hundred men and few soldiers could afford to resort to prostitution.

In some ways the slaves on the plantations were better off than the soldiers – at least they had developed an immunity to yellow fever. Occasionally, with the connivance of one of them, a group of soldiers would break into a sugar plantation and drink themselves into a stupor. In these circumstances it was not surprising that the men fell victim to fever about once in every sixteen months. The illness usually lasted for three months and killed a quarter of its victims. Barry faced her first outbreak at Stoney Hill, a military station nine miles from Kingston in August 1831. Even her determined efforts could not defeat the virulent disease. And those years of hard work in the gruelling sun undoubtedly aged her, both physically and mentally. She was only thirty-two but she already looked 'withered and old'.

At Christmas 1831 the little doctor with her high-heeled boots, her reddish hair (dyed, it was whispered), was faced with a situation that taxed her even more. The planters enjoyed good living all the year round. They held huge banquets with groaning tables of meats, washed down with bottles of foreign wine and rum, while the slaves fed on salt fish and salt pork. But at Christmas even the slaves enjoyed a respite from the long hours of working in the fields, cutting the sugar cane or grinding and boiling it, with the overseer standing over them with a cartwhip. For three whole days they were petted and feasted by the planters. Each one received an individual present. They were egged on to stage pageants in costume to amuse the whites and allowed to hold dances amongst themselves. Elaborate balls for white men and coloured women were held, so that mistresses could be chosen, and the slaves were officially allowed to taste the rum and liquor from the plantation distilleries.

In 1831 Christmas Day fell on a Sunday. On the day after Boxing Day the slaves were expected to turn up for work and lose one of their days of freedom. That missing free day incensed them: nine-tenths of the slaves of the parish of Trelawny, in the north-west of Jamaica, refused to work. Passive resistance was their leaders' intention, but before the day was out the slaves broke into a rum store and 'the devil got into their heads'. They set fire to mansion houses and sugar works. For miles the sky was 'lit up with a lurid glare'.

Since there was no permanent white barracks in this mountainous and wooded part of the island, a local coloured militia, led by a planter, was called out to quash the rising. The force was ill-equipped and badly led, and the commander, Colonel Gignon, retreated before the rebels on 29th December, leaving the rest of the country in the hands of the slaves. On New Year's Day regular troops landed under the command of Sir Willoughby Cotton, an officer more at home in the drawing-rooms of fashionable London, where he enjoyed a reputation as a wit and *bon viveur*, than in the steaming forests of Jamaica.

'I served under Sir Willoughby Cotton during the Rebellion and burning of the plantations by the negroes', Barry commented tersely in an official memorandum on her service. This was her first experience of field work in charge of the health of the troops.

Four days after the troops landed, the Governor had the situation under control. Martial law ceased. The redcoats with their guns had quickly quelled the rebels armed only with knives and stones. Ten white men and nearly 400 black slaves were killed in the fighting. Considering that about 50 000 slaves had rebelled, the loss of life to the white Colonists was relatively small. Nevertheless the slaves were punished savagely: about 100 Negroes were shot, and another 100 'severely flogged'. One woman slave, condemned to death, was spared – no doubt because she was pregnant. Over £80 000 worth of damage was done to over 100 plantations, and whole settlements were razed to the ground. After the rising and the damage to their fine estates, the planters felt the need for military protection. As a result the appallingly unhealthy station at Montego Bay was reopened, and the soldiers died of dysentery and fever to keep the wealthy estate owners safe from harm.

The barracks were sited in the town, cut off from sea breezes by surrounding mountains, and the heat was intense – the thermometer never fell below the nineties. Even the residents scarcely passed a season without serious illness. Several times in the past it had been necessary to close down the barracks and withdraw the troops because there were no men left on their feet. All Barry could do was to reopen the hospital, a dank stone building, without verandahs or balconies and impose her usual régime of rigorous cleanliness. Nevertheless in 1832 forty-four of the garrison of 123 men stationed at Montego Bay died.

Because of the emergency other outposts in the north and east of the island were reopened; they too took their toll. At the fort at Buff's Bay there were seven dead out of a total of twenty-five; at Manchioneal not one man was left on duty; the whole force had succumbed to fever, and at Chapel Town there were fourteen deaths in six months. These bleak figures cover a terrible waste of life, and Barry, with her feeling for the ordinary soldier, must have suffered indignation and wretchedness. The Director General of the Army Medical Department was advised in a report sent home that outposts in these very unhealthy stations could not be manned without 'a great sacrifice to life'. The advice was ignored. When it came to the Army in peacetime politicians at home were ignorant or indifferent. Cuts in defence spending were always popular in Parliament and even liberals and radicals, so concerned about slavery, were quick to exploit the support these economies carried. Nor were the staff at the Horse Guards much better. They were Wellington's men, officers who had fought at Waterloo and still lived in the past. They simply did not understand the needs of an army stationed hundreds of miles away in the tropics.

In her sixteen years of army service Barry had seen more cruelty and privation than most men of her age and education would ever see. Certainly she knew more about the troops' lives than the general staff. She met death almost daily as a doctor, senseless death that could have been prevented by giving the troops decent living conditions. But one branch of the army administration was beginning to acknowledge the terrible waste of men through disease. The head of the Army Medical Department, Sir James McGrigor, pointed out in a memorandum in 1833 that army doctors needed special skills that 'even the examinations of the College of Physicians and the College of Surgeons do not extend to': they required a knowledge of tropical illness and the capacity to detect the 'feigned diseases of soldiers'.

Any unfortunate soldier who feigned illness with Dr Barry would gain short shrift. Though compassionate with real sufferers, she was impatient and short-tempered with those she felt were wasting her time.

She was now most often to be found at the Up Park Camp, two miles north of Kingston, where she lived in the Colonel's quarters. The barracks at Up Park were airy and the hospital, one storey high, had a balcony all round. Off duty, she was to be seen driving round the island in her brougham dressed in a blue frock-coat with a black silk stock – immaculately turned out as usual.

Living alone, as she did, with no one to share the horrors she encountered, unable to relax completely until she was by herself, it is hardly surprising that she became more eccentric and unlike her fellow officers. Writing after her death, a former colleague, General Chamberlayne, remembered with some insight that in Jamaica Barry was 'rather bombastic in speech and repellent in manner, but kind and anxious to do good to those who were never likely to become intrusive or familiar or troublesome to her'. Her colleagues remarked that she had 'a dislike of medical men' (too many past quarrels, and a fear of detection perhaps?), and a 'queer fondness for animals'. Increasingly she was to find an outlet for her affection with animals who could be relied upon never to blab.

A fellow officer, Colonel R. Wilson, remembered dining with Barry at General Ashmore's where she was a frequent guest. As usual she was the source of some malicious fun for her fellow officers.

We were all much amused at the outrageous stories she used to tell, making herself out to be quite a lady-killer . . . at balls or parties she was certain to tack herself on to the finest and best-looking women in the room . . . yet like most women she loved attending weddings, christenings etc.

The comments were made after Barry's death, when the scandal of her sex was known, therefore they must be regarded with some reservation. However, there is no doubt that Barry fitted uncomfortably into the officers' world. She was isolated from her colleagues by her fastidious tastes. Hers was a dry sarcastic wit which sprang from intellectual interests far beyond the understanding of most of the officers of the day. As General Chamberlayne remarked, her conversation was superior to that usually heard in the mess. She could not compete in the talk of gambling and horses, yet here, as at the Cape, she cultivated her reputation as a womanizer. One officer even complained that she always visited his wife late in the evening when he was out. Did her gallantry provide her with an excuse to seek out feminine society while proving to the world how manly she was?

Barry was still in Jamaica in August 1834, when Parliament passed an Act banning slavery. The attitude of the planters and of the House of Assembly towards the new legislation must have appalled her. According to Sir Lionel Smith, the Governor, the planters 'would be delighted to get up an insurrection for the pleasure of destroying the negroes and missionaries. They are quite mad.'

In April 1835, when Barry was home on leave, the Marquess of Sligo, in a letter to the Army Medical Department, observed that patients recovered more quickly under local doctors than under the military. The general opinion, wrote the Marquess from Jamaica was that a large permanent medical staff was needed at big general hospitals. On arrival, he added, all regimental surgeons should be compelled to attend the hospital and the local practitioners should be invited to practise there. The recommendations sounded eminently sensible; they also have the ring of Dr James Barry. Plainly her work had not been entirely fruitless.

For four years Dr Barry had remained out of the news. When she came home on leave in February 1835 it was officially and honourably, after a gruelling four years' service. London must have seemed a changed city to her. Horse-drawn omnibuses carried passengers from the East to the West End; steamboats plied to and from Greenwich every half an hour; streets were brighter and more and more private houses were lit by gas.

Fashions for women were elaborate: bustles and bonnets, whalebone bodices, muffs and ribbons, and sweeping skirts. After twenty years of fighting disease, facing squalor and taking command Barry could hardly have envied the life of a demure Victorian spinster. Yet perhaps she hankered after another kind of life – almost certainly she must have sometimes longed to be a private person, a woman able to express her femininity.

As far as we know, she separated her life into two compartments: her childhood and adolescence were cut off completely from her army career. If her family and relatives were still alive, then she had lost touch with them during her gruelling years in the service. No family correspondence exists. Contact with her mother and elder sister must have been extremely tenuous, and no evidence remains to suggest visits or family reunions. Her masquerade forced her to live her daily life in unimaginable loneliness. On leave she visited those friends whom she had first met in the service – such as Vice-Admiral Sir Jahleel Brenton, who had recently been appointed Governor of Greenwich Hospital. Her link with the Beaufort family remained constant.

Fitzroy Somerset, then Secretary at the Horse Guards, almost certainly influenced the posting to her next appointment. It was an unusual one: she was ordered to St Helena to take charge of both the civilian and military wings of the regimental hospitals. With her record of vigorous reform and her reputation for making trouble at the Cape the posting must have been carefully thought out. Sir James McGrigor, who was Wellington's Medical Officer during the Peninsular War, prided himself on knowing his officers well, and promoting them on the grounds of length of service, professional character and experience.

From Barry's point of view it was a tricky appointment. St Helena was in a state of transition. The island had prospered under the Royal East India Company's rule until two years previously, when it had been ceded to the Crown. The Company had departed, taking with them their three garrisons, their medical men and most of the potential for wealth on the island.

Barry left London on the 18th of April, 1836 with her servant and joined the ship, the *Lord William Bentinck*, East Indiaman, off Deal six days later. On board she met an old friend, Sir Andries Stockenstrom, a magistrate whom she had known nineteen years earlier at the Cape. The ship took seventy-four days to reach Table Bay and the voyage was 'unpleasant and protracted'. On the 8th of May an epidemic of smallpox broke out on board and in his account Sir Andries noted that 'one poor woman died and was immediately buried' and 'there were five cases in all'.

When the ship landed at the Cape the most rigorous measures were taken by the health authorities to prevent the spread of smallpox. Clothing and bedding were burnt, letters fumigated and the passengers were forced to spend six weeks in a temporary hospital, known as a lazaretto, at the Chavonnes battery. Worst of all, from Barry's point of view, no dogs or cats were allowed ashore.

She objected vehemently, and suggested an acceptable solution. Psyche, she proposed, should be allowed to swim ashore, then be washed in disinfected fluid and kept chained away from other dogs. The Governor seemed disposed to agree.

But Barry's other property received scant courtesy. In a letter to the Governor dated 23rd of August, 1836, she wrote:

My bedding was burnt, my linen, a large quantity requisite in a long voyage, steeped in chloride of lime until so decimated that it fell to rags in washing, three pillows of a particular description necessary to me under the peculiar circumstances in which severe accidents have placed me which cost fifteen guineas each were wantonly and against my strongest remonstrance seized and destroyed.

No record exists of any accident which could explain why Barry needed special pillows. But in South Africa and in other stations there were rumours that she wrapped herself in towels. presumably she used them to pad out her shoulders. Were they also used, perhaps, during menstruation?

She put in a claim for her property, 'disposed of without positive necessity', for forty-six days' board and lodging and for the difference between her pay in quarantine and at St Helena. The total came to £212. 3s.

There is no evidence that it was paid. The Secretary to the

Government at the Cape remarked that it was 'the most extraordinary claim he had ever seen'.

James Barry Munnik, her godson, recalled after her death that he saw her almost daily while she waited in quarantine, but we hear no more of her until her arrival on the tiny island of St Helena in September 1836. Within two months she was in trouble.

8

Not Guilty on My Honour

In the second half of the nineteenth century St Helena was to become an important coaling station in the British Navy, but when Barry arrived there in 1836 the island, with its white-washed Georgian houses, pine trees and camellias, was a cut off little world, surrounded by rugged hills and a band of desolate black rocks. In Jamestown, the capital, the English settlers led prosperous lives in comfortable colonial style until the Royal East India Company moved out, when many of the younger men left the island to find new employment, abandoning their womenfolk. However, those settlers who remained continued to dine out, attend balls, and wait for a sign of news from home, for a sail in the blue, blue sea. In the garrison town the Governor reigned supreme and the officers of the Army, redcoated and resplendent, led the social life of the Colony.

As Principal Medical Officer, Barry lived in comfort in a pretty cottage in Jamestown, and enjoyed the English flowers and the delicious fruits of the island: peaches and plums, grapes and passion fruit and above all mangoes. Since she was a vegetarian and abhorred apples and potatoes ('filthy roots', she called them) the abundance of tropical fruits provided her with a delightful daily diet.

But in 1836 there was an acute shortage of manpower and doctors on St Helena, and for all its camellia charm, Barry saw the other side of the colonists' world. Her patients included 'paupers, prisoners and convicts; lascars and invalids of the East India Company, Bendas and seamen from Dutch, French and American' ships.

She plunged into work with her usual energy. Many patients were suffering from scurvy; others from accidents; some even needed 'capital operations'. She held a clinic every day at the dispensary, between 2 and 3 p.m., and prescribed for the paupers. She also visited the sick in prison and set up a vaccination system, an important innovation in a colony 'where ships touch for water from many parts of the world'. Disease travelled with crew, passengers and the rats that scuttled ashore, which placed the inhabitants of a seaport at special risk. In the past a bundle of washing taken in from a ship infected with measles had caused the loss of many lives at St Helena.

Before long she had concerned herself with the soldiers' diet. She was convinced that dysentery, so common among the troops, was due to lack of fresh food. She endorsed the findings of a medical board which recommended replacing the soldiers' daily diet – a pound of salt beef or salt pork (plus a pound of bread) washed down with a pint of Cape wine – for two days of fresh food per week with the right to exchange the salt meat or fish for vegetables, an innovation which proved important in combating gastric diseases. As a vegetarian Barry valued fruits and vegetables highly. Her batman, a Mr McCosh, alleged that she gave her meat ration to her dog – a ration the troops could rarely afford. But although she was also a teetotaller by the St Helena days, she felt bound to point out the 'eminent utility' of Cape wine as an antidote to scurvy.

For once she was tolerably satisfied with the hospital arrangements for the military, and described the regimental hospital, under the direction of Assistant Surgeon Eddie as 'clean and well arranged'. She also praised Surgeon Eddie for his 'zeal, ability and attention' in directing it. It was to his care that Barry attributed the decline in the death rate among his patients. For if most people remember Dr Barry for her scathing pen and sardonic criticism, she could be generous to colleagues who upheld her standards.

But within a week of her arrival she was beside herself with anger at the 'confused and disgusting' state of the civil section of the hospital (the hospital building was divided into two sections, one for the military, the other for civilians). Men and women, prostitutes and soldiers crowded the wards. With the departure of the Royal East India Company, the rate of venereal disease had increased alarmingly in an island where brothels and drinking houses had always existed for the 'inferior part of the fleet'. Many women left stranded by men of the Company had turned to prostitution as their only means of livelihood.

Barry exploded at 'the disgusting circumstance of male attendants on the female patients with syphilitic and other diseases – and of course the greatest irregularities – I immediately hired a respectable woman of colour as matron and requested the military chaplain to visit the civil side of the hospital'.

As usual Barry was outstandingly modern. The concept of a respectable woman taking to nursing, a profession usually embraced by 'fallen' or drunken women, was one that Florence Nightingale is said to have introduced. Yet, quite naturally, almost twenty years before the Crimean War, Barry employed a coloured matron in her hospital at St Helena.

Within a month of arriving, she had cajoled the Governor, Major-General Middlemore, into consenting to convert an empty building, close to the regimental hospital (nicknamed 'The Brewery'), to be equipped as an entirely separate civilian hospital. She wanted 'one portion for the reception of females and the other for maniacs who are in an awfully neglected state'. In St Helena, as at the Cape, Barry showed a particular, and in the circumstances a very natural, interest in the plight of women in institutions. But her insistent and repeated demands for reform, couched in language which was undiplomatic to say the least, were, once again, to prove damaging to her career.

Her duties on St Helena were exceptionally heavy. As well as superintending the civilian wing of the hospital, she was responsible for the health of the garrison and the various working parties scattered about the island. She also looked after the officers and their families. And then there was all the paper work: filling in 'endless forms and returns and reports' to the War Office, and coping with medical boards and hospital arrangements.

Before long she was involved in a blazing row with the Commissariat. This department, staffed mainly by civilians and under the direct control of the Treasury, rather than the Secretary at War, organized supplies for the Army. These officials were as hidebound and obstreperous in supplying the hospital at St Helena in 1836 as they were in providing for the medical needs of the troops in the Crimea, nearly twenty years later. Since however, it was a fight about an obscure peacetime hospital, Barry – unlike Florence Nightingale – did not win any glory.

The quarrel began when Barry asked the Assistant Commissary General, a Mr W. Knowles, to furnish both the military and civilian wings of the hospital with supplies. To buy goods wholesale for both hospitals would work out more cheaply she pointed out sensibly. He refused point-blank: the civilian sick were not his responsibility.

She also asked him to supply the military wing of the hospital with its full quota of provisions. (Before her arrival the Commissariat had supplied only the basics: bread, meat, coals and candles. Other articles needed, such as sago, salt, milk, tea, sugar, and so on, had been bought and paid for by the Medical Officer.)

Barry would not be a party to this irregular arrangement although it saved the Commissariat work. She had been carefully instructed in her duties before she left England and the rule required the Commissariat to buy every article asked for. 'Dr Barry did not see the slightest reason for a deviation from either the letter or the spirit of the rule.'

She also pointed out that in her orders she had been asked to make separate estimates of requisitions for supplies to the troops and civilian population, but 'no distinction is made in the mode of obtaining supplies'. She added that although the duties of supplying the civilian wing were not laid down specifically as part of the Assistant Commissary General's duties, it was her opinion 'that the intentions of the Lords of the Treasury are to be supplied to all hospitals under the charge of military medical men'. Once again Barry was taking on the responsibility of telling other people where their duty lay. Mr Knowles insisted that the services she wanted him to undertake were 'strictly of a civil nature under the control of the civil Government', and ought to be defrayed not from the military chest – but out of the funds of the colony: 'I can have no control whatever over such expenditure.'

Since the Ordnance Department of the army was providing for the needs of the civilian wing, there must have been some reason for the Assistant Commissary's objection. Perhaps he was loath to take orders from a new odd-looking officer, who seemed only to want to give him more work. Perhaps he disliked innovation. Whatever it was, Barry urged Mr Knowles most courteously to reconsider his decision 'in the hopes of averting the necessity of a reference home'.

He refused again. That settled it. Barry took the unprecedented step of writing direct to the Secretary at War.

In her letter she explained the problem, quoted chapter and verse of the regulations for the management of hospitals on foreign stations, and sent a copy of the correspondence between Knowles and herself. She added disdainfully: 'It will appear unnecessary to comment on the total absence of all rational objection on the part of the Commissariat here to further the ends of the service.' She had, of course, a clerk to copy her letter and it was thanks to him, perhaps, that news of its existence leaked out. On a small island, rumour travels fast and soon all the senior officials and the Governor had heard of her extraordinary action – an action which must, to them, have seemed high-handed and threatening in the extreme.

On November the 13th, 1836, three days after she had drafted the letter Barry was 'bathing in the morning' at her residence

> when my servant told me that Major Barnes [the Town Major] wanted me immediately.
>
> I asked him to wait a moment, I put on my dressing gown and he said, 'I am sorry, Barry, I have bad news for you.' I was seized with agitation and asked if a ship had arrived. He said 'No. I am come to put you in arrest' and he produced the orders . . . I thought he was mad – I stared at him.

With extraordinary presence of mind, Barry asked the Town Major whether the General of the Garrison was aware that she was to be arrested. He was not.

> I of course spurned the idea of such a thing and saying I could not acknowledge his authority, I immediately draped and proceeded to Town with a view to going directly to the General to report the thing and state that as Principal Medical Officer, I was entitled to his protection.

Barry went out in the carriage of a friend, a Mr Solomon, her sword by her side, and drove straight to the Governor's residence, Plantation House. On her way there she was intercepted. The Town Major, on horseback, stopped her, saying he had the Governor's authority. She ordered the carriage home and sat down to write a formal protest. Town Major Barnes called again, this time officially to place her under arrest.

I asked Major Barnes what I should do . . . I had never been in arrest . . . I had patients of the greatest importance, one dying, two dead at the hospital.

Town Major Barnes admitted that he knew about her patients, but insisted that she must not stir. Protocol, in the Colonies, took precedence even over matters of life and death. As in Cape Town, she was battling with petty officials who were concerned to uphold the establishment which tolerated their accommodation within it. Barry had sinned against the system – and that was unforgivable. She was court-martialled; the charge: 'conduct unbecoming to an officer and a gentleman'. After a masquerade as a man lasting twenty years could anything be more ludicrous?

Under arrest, confined to her home, 'disgraced', Barry nevertheless displayed tremendous courage. On the 15th of November she took the occasion to remind the Governor of the 'confused and disgusting' arrangements in the civilian wing, where venereal disease among the troops was rampant, and the wards were packed with prostitutes, soldiers, paupers and seamen. She urgently requested that the separate building for females and maniacs be made ready. 'We shall be at a loss to accommodate even the troops in the event of accident or increase of disease in the Garrison', she warned.

One gets the feeling that by carrying on with her work, she held herself in check. Nevertheless the strain on her must have been overwhelming: once again she was exposed to the public view and an object of gossip and rumour.

The court proceedings were farcical, and the level of argument pathetic. 'Not guilty on my Honour' was Barry's plea; she conducted her own defence. During the hearing Assistant Commissary Knowles acknowledged that he was *accusing* Barry as a *defence* of himself. He demanded 'an absolute and unqualified acquittal of the accusation alleged against me to the Secretary at War' from the Court. Barry had apparently insulted his pride. 'The prisoner will tell you that I am only a Warrant Officer. I am the same rank as the prisoner, comparable to a Captain in the Army. My commission was in 1816. His was in 1827.' (An indisputable fact which merely revealed that Assistant Commissary Knowles had not received promotion in twenty years!)

Barry stood up excellently to the necessarily weak prosecution. 'It was', she suggested 'probably the first instance of an officer being brought to trial for the performance of his duty.'

But Mr Knowles did make one point which seems unanswerable. 'Are the Lords of the Treasury', he asked 'to be troubled in disproving the complaints of Dr Barry?' She did, throughout her career, involve the authorities, local and at home, in a weight of correspondence and paper work. Her ambiguous role in life led her to justify herself and her position whenever she felt threatened.

On the third day of her trial a friend came to the courtroom to announce that Dr Barry was 'very unwell' and would like to be permitted half an hour's repose. Apart from the ordeal of defending herself in public, wasting her time on such ridiculous charges must have exasperated her almost beyond endurance. The trial lasted a fortnight and revealed yet more about the hidden workings of the Colony's administration. Although asked by both Barry and the Court to testify, the Governor, Major-General Middlemore, refused. It became clear during the proceedings that Knowles had shown the Governor a copy of some of the correspondence about the civilian wing of the hospital, although the Assistant Commissary vehemently denied it. Barry testified that she had been to see the Governor about the hospital and while she was there, General Middlemore 'drew out his table drawer saying "I have had correspondence with Knowles on the subject of Hospitals". The Governor took out the letter and a private note, beginning with "My dear General" – I looked no further – a gentleman ought not to do so.' This quixotic recourse to the ideal of gentlemanly behaviour was a constant theme in one guise or another, in Barry's life. It always led her into trouble: gentlemen, alas, lied, gossiped and intrigued. Barry's letter had been copied and copied until it had been distorted almost beyond recognition.

Faced with these machinations Barry was indiscreet. Assistant Commissary Knowles was 'known to possess a certain influence with the Governor', she said in Court. 'It is equally notorious that he had been in personal communication with His Excellency since the adjournment.'

This may have been true, but it was unwise of Barry to mention the matter. Knowles accused her, with some justification, in his closing speech of 'blinking and cloaking the original charge and, as it were, smothering it with a host of extraneous rubbish'.

In her final plea to the Court, Barry preferred 'not to enter into a dissertation on the mental and bodily injury inflicted on a delicate constitution by the vexatious proceedings'. In a seemingly irrelevant aside, she told the Court that 'at the Cape of Good Hope, the late Lord Charles Somerset, the Governor of that Colony, suffered much in mind and body from garbled statements from his persecutors, through which he lost his life but saved his honour'. (It is significant that under stress Barry instinctively referred to Lord Charles Somerset.) And she added another personal note; 'When I was a boy', she told the Court, 'I was told that when I began a story, to begin at the beginning and continue to the end . . .' Had she, after over twenty-five years of masquerading as a man, begun to believe that she belonged to the 'gentlemanly sex'? 'If for a single instant', she said in her defence, 'I could imagine I have lost sight of the character of a gentleman I should have spared this or any other tribunal the task of investigating my conduct.'

The Court, having 'maturely weighed and considered the evidence', found that the prisoner, James Barry, wrote the letter – but was justified in so doing. She was fully and honourably acquitted – officially at least – and allowed to return to her duties.

But her difficulties were not over yet. The Governor, General Middlemore, sent the proceedings to Fitzroy Somerset accompanied by a letter in which he attempted to clear himself and blame Barry.

The Major General Commanding regrets that in the proceedings . . . so much extraneous and irrelevant matter has been introduced [*Knowles's very words!*]. *Likewise certain accusations which are*

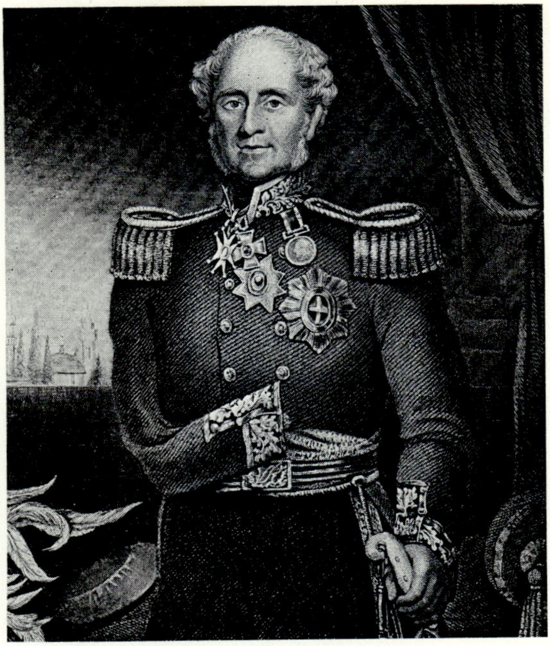

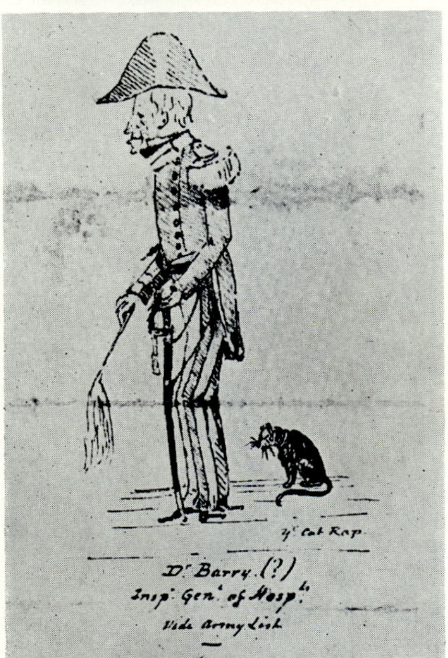

(Above) *Fitzroy Somerset, later Lord Raglan, a discreet influence on Barry's military career.*

A pen drawing of Barry, in the uniform of Deputy Inspector General of Hospitals, with Psyche (?) and horse-hair whip. The caricature is attributed to Edward Lear who was staying in Corfu at the time Barry was serving there.

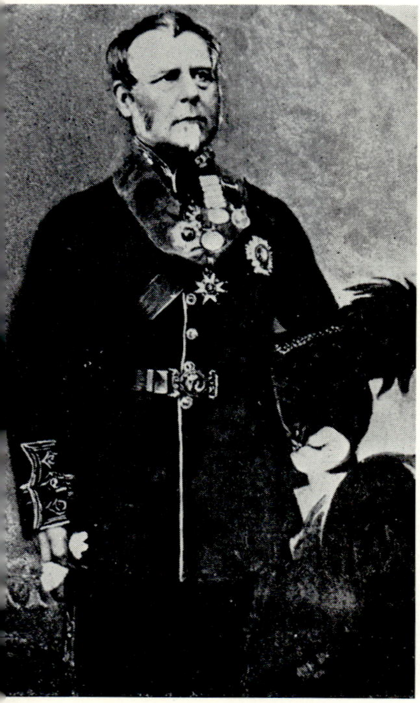

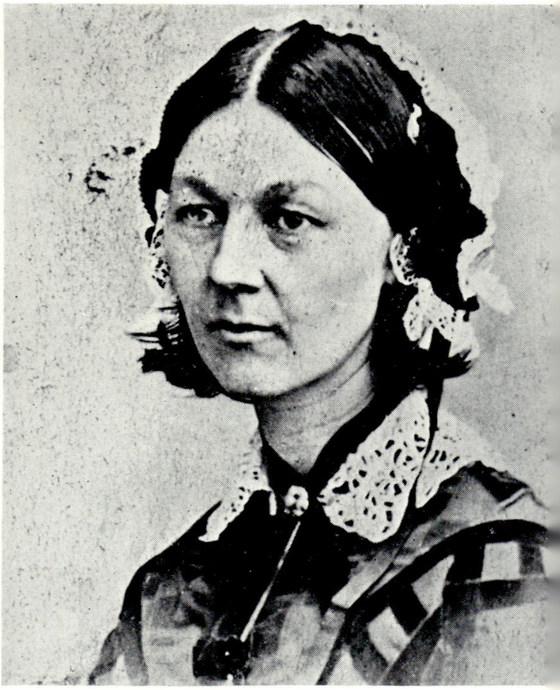

(Above left) *Sir John Hall, Inspector General of Hospitals in the Crimea, described by Florence Nightingale as 'Knight of the Crimean Burial Grounds'.*

(Above right) *Florence Nightingale*

Embarkation of sick and wounded soldiers at Balaclava, many of whom were nursed back to health by Barry in Corfu.

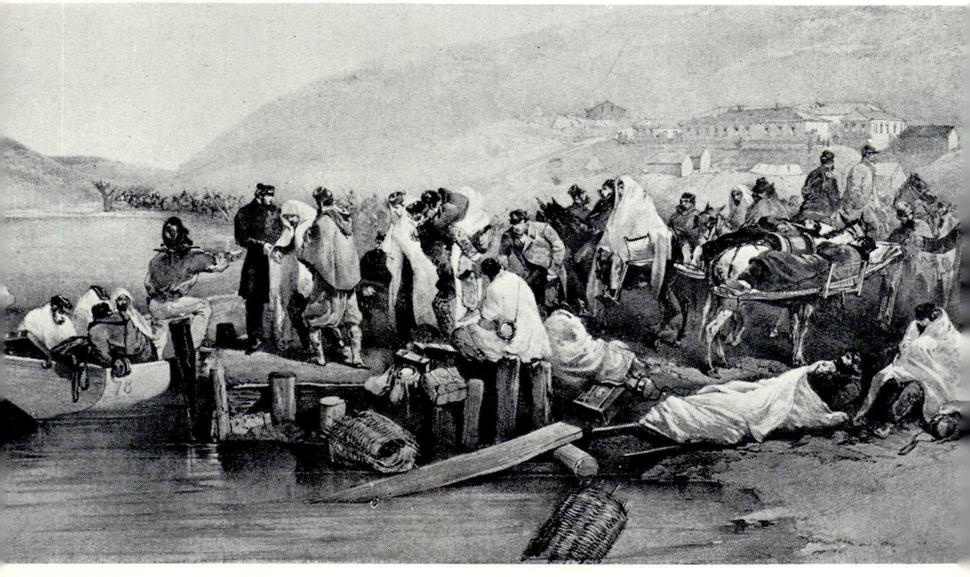

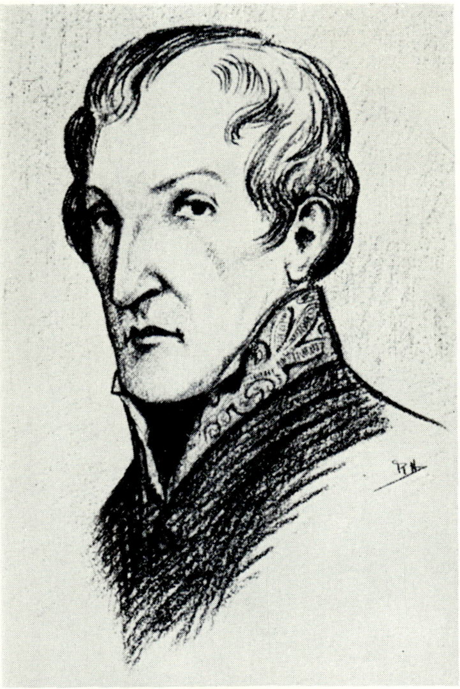

A pencil sketch of Barry as Inspector General of the Army Medical Department, her last appointment.

(Below) *The street in Montreal where Dr Barry lived during her posting as Inspector General. The severe winter of 1858 ended her career.*

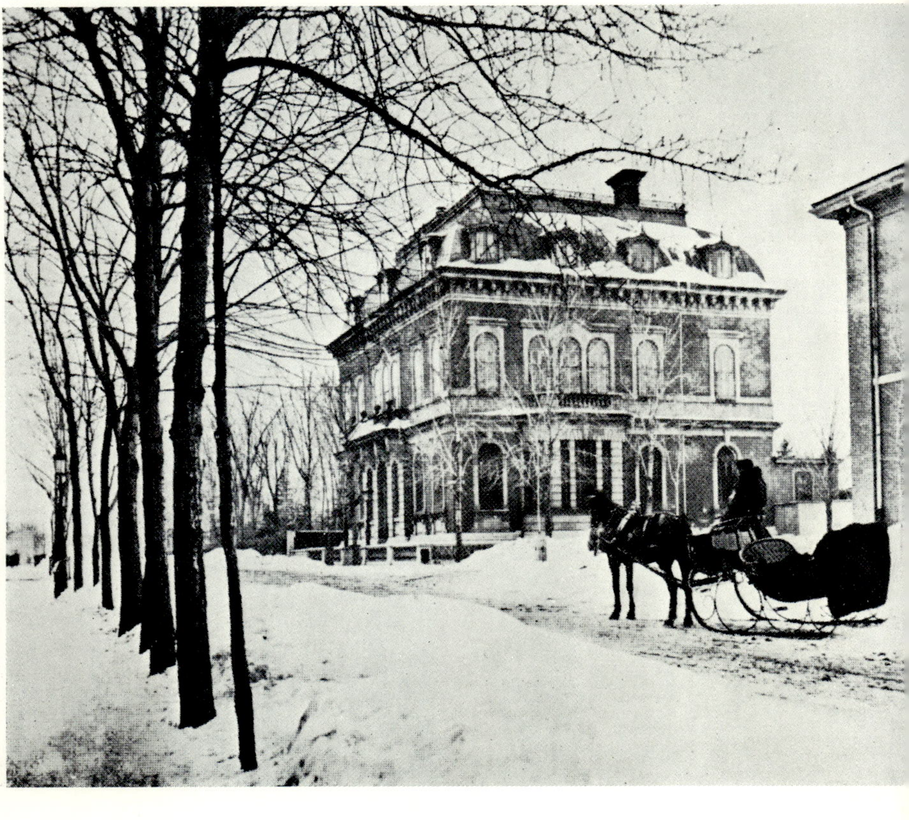

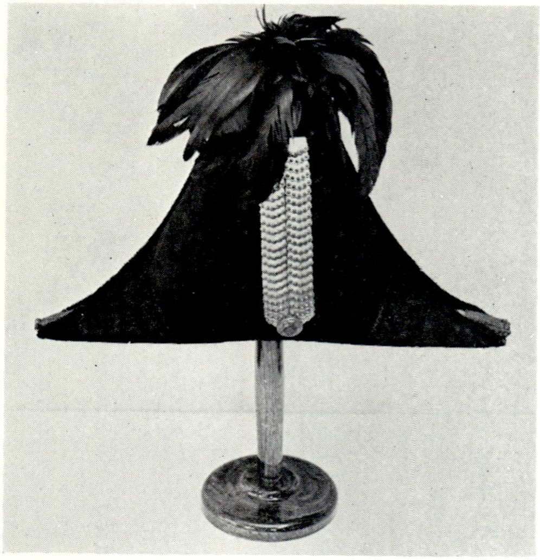

Barry's cocked hat, part of the full-dress uniform of an Inspector General.

Her grave at Kensal Green Cemetery. The stone is now flattened and the plot overgrown.

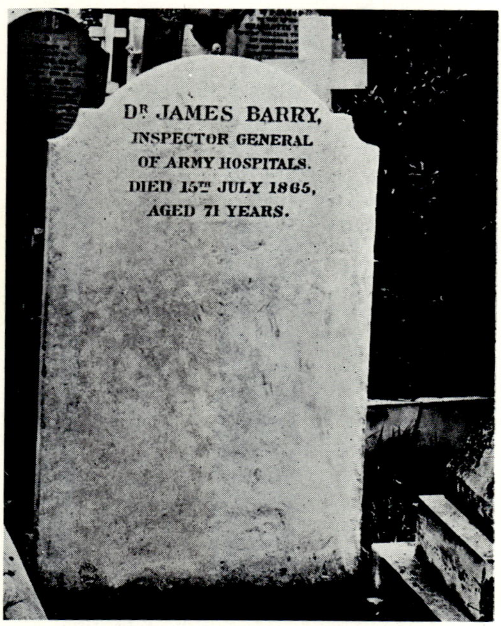
DR JAMES BARRY,
INSPECTOR GENERAL
OF ARMY HOSPITALS.
DIED 15TH JULY 1865,
AGED 71 YEARS.

calculated to reflect on the Major General Commanding in declining to attend in Evidence in the above Trial, especially as his evidence did not relate to the charge.

Fitzroy Somerset duly forwarded the proceedings to the Judge Advocate General.

The authorities at home were coming to recognize that wherever Dr Barry went she caused trouble in one way or another. Yet in St Helena, as at the Cape, Barry had succeeded in changing the system at a cost to her career. She could not resist writing a triumphant little note attached to the verdict. 'The Lords Commissioners of H.M. Treasury ordered the Commissariat Department to provide for the civilian wing of the hospital by contract, the same as for the Military, by which means the Government saved considerably and the patients were better provided for.'

Predictably, before long, the Principal Medical Officer was involved in yet another row. This time it was a question of pay. For the year she was due to receive £274. 5s. plus £38. 12s. forage for her horse, a sum which included her civil, as well as her army, pay. However she received her full salary only once – during her first month on the island. Knowles lay behind this fresh irritation. From the time of their conflict, he had looked for an excuse to spite her and by delving into past records he had managed to find one. Triumphantly he pointed out to the Governor that medical officers who treated civilians were not entitled to an extra allowance, and should refund the 'overplus'.

General Middlemore (who was in debt to the Government at home and always anxious to placate them) wrote to Lord Glenelg at the Colonial Office, confessing his 'grievous error' in paying medical officers the extra allowance and asking for a decision for the future. The answer was a foregone conclusion. The Army in peacetime was unpopular and any money that could be saved was welcome.

Barry wrote to protest – on behalf of her juniors, Assistant Surgeon Hopkins and Apothecary Courtney, as well as herself. She pointed out the justice of their claims; other officers in the command received extra pay for civilian work – a Captain Alexander of the Engineers, for example, received an extra 10s.

a day; Town Major Barnes had an extra 10s. per day, and the Military Chaplain, Mr Helps, received £250 a year extra. In fact any military officer who carried out civilian duties was duly compensated.

Letters flew back and forth from Sir James McGrigor, who upheld his staff's claim for extra pay, to the Lords of the Treasury and from the Treasury to the Under Secretary of the Colonial Department. Both Sir James McGrigor and Lord Fitzroy Somerset sought to further Barry's claim but without success. Barry herself campaigned tirelessly for three years. She was tenacious by nature, and whether she was battling for better conditions for the underprivileged or for fair compensation for herself and her fellow officers, she loathed giving in.

Meanwhile her urgent request for a separate civilian hospital, put in nine months earlier, seemed at last to be making some headway with the authorities. In June 1837 General Middlemore finally asked for an estimate for converting the empty Government building, and the total outlay for the hospital for civil patients, 'especially females', was assessed at £167. 18s. 4d. However Barry was never to see it built.

After her court martial her life on St Helena held very few bright moments and to receive a letter from her godson, James Barry Munnik, the little boy she had delivered eleven years earlier must have been a welcome reminder of a happy time. In December 1837 she wrote one of the few personal letters that still survive. Today it is treasured in a frame by Mrs Treleaven (formerly Mrs James Barry Munnik).

My dear James Barry

I was much pleased with your letter and it was well written and it does you and your master great credit. I should have written to you before but I hoped your watch would have arrived from England. I expect it daily – you have a young friend of mine Mr Baker at your school.

I hope you and he are friends. Write to me by every opportunity. Remember me most kindly to your father and to Mrs Sandenberg and Basham and his Lady to my dear old friend his mother, Mrs Cloete. I trust she is quite well.

I have not time to say more than God bless my Dear Boy and prosper you.

James Barry

The watch, so lovingly ordered, never arrived. The reason, according to family tradition, is that the boy James Barry wrote to his godparent innocently reporting that 'people are talking about you and saying that you look rather like a lady'. Barry put her guard up and did not reply to that letter.

With the new year Governor Middlemore began a campaign to have her recalled. Ever since the court martial he had distrusted her. She was an embarrassment to his rule, her demands for reform would involve him in extra expense and since he was in debt to the Government, that would be awkward. All in all he would be glad to be rid of her.

He wrote to Lord Glenelg, Secretary of State for the Colonies:

I have to regret that Dr James Barry has so conducted himself that I have ordered him home under arrest. The proceedings of a Court of Inquiry with various documents relative to Dr James Barry's conduct have been transmitted for the Commander-in-Chief's information and guidance, by the London, *in which ship Dr James Barry embarked.*

Once again Barry had been victimized by officials smarting under her caustic tongue and her high-handed mode of achieving reform. This time, however, there was no protector to suspend the sentence.

An eyewitness reported Barry's departure from the island with her pony, her black servant and her poodle:

On one of those still, sultry mornings peculiar to the tropics, the measured steps of the doctor's pony woke up the echoes of the valley. Then came the P.M.O. looking faded and crestfallen. He was in plain clothes. He had shrunk away wonderfully. His blue jacket hung loosely about him and his white trousers were a world too wide. The veil garnishing his broad straw hat covered his face and he carried the inevitable umbrella over his head so that it saved him from the general gaze. The street was deserted but other eyes than the writer's looked on the group through the Venetian blinds. No sentry presented arms at the gates and the familiar quartet proceeded unnoticed along the lines to the ship's boat in waiting.

As at the Cape, it is clear that for those patients she had tended, Barry's departure meant renewed hardship. Soon the Governor was reporting that the 'sick poor of the island' were neglected and the chaplain in a letter to the church warden in that year, remarked on their 'deplorable state'.

Whatever passed between Barry, McGrigor and Fitzroy Somerset in London, is off the record. No trace of the documents of the Court of Inquiry survives in the War Office files either. The only fact that emerges is that by August 1838, Dr Barry, far from being demoted, was fighting to get back the pay due to her for what Sir James himself described as 'heavy Colonial duties in St Helena'.

She wrote to Lord Glenelg, pressing her claim to her pay for civil duties, from her house in St James's.

Permit me here my Lord to observe, that having to establish some system, everything being in a most confused and disgusting state so far as the Military and Civil Hospitals were concerned on my arrival – it required great exertion and much ungracious and painful duties fell to my lot – from which although I have personally heavily suffered – yet I am proud to say the service has benefitted considerably.

Other officers on the command received extra pay for civilian duties, and she ended her letter by reiterating, 'on the same grounds if not stronger', her right to similar consideration.

A note on the back of her letter remarks that 'it is impossible to entertain a claim for services of this nature unless it be preferred according to the established course of business'. These delaying tactics deferred her claim to her old enemy, General Middlemore, who set up a Medical Board to consider it.

The Board was made up of the Governor's men: Mr Courtney, the new Principal Medical Officer (appointed on Barry's departure, but without the Government's approval), Assistant Surgeon McClaren and Assistant Surgeon Eddie; they were all junior to Barry.

Even allowing for two or three months' postal delay it took a long time to assemble the Board, and not until February 25th 1839 did they finally meet. The document they produced is remarkable.

The officers of the Board acknowledged that Barry had performed various civil duties efficiently, but rebuked her for not pointing out 'the important services of Assistant Staff Surgeon Hopkins in the Civil Hospital and of Mr Courtney [the President of the Board], Apothecary to the Forces in the Dispensary'. (They did not see fit to add that Dr Barry had originally made her claim on behalf of Staff Surgeon Hopkins and Mr Courtney as well as herself.)

With almost maidenly demureness, the report continued:

The board now approaches an extremely delicate and painful part of its duty viz., a becoming notice of Dr James Barry's extraordinary conduct in endeavouring apparently to augment the assumed value of his own service by something stronger than mere disparagement of the others as evinced in his allegation of the 'confused and disgusting' state in which he found the hospital.

The Board is willing to hope for the sake of truth and candour that Dr James Barry might possibly only have intended an allusion to the defective state of the accommodation and not a reflection on the Administration of the duties of the hospital and the Board feels happily relieved from all necessity for further comment by the impossibility of its being believed that H.E. Major-General Middlemore or Lt. Colonel Anderson, Commanding the 91st Regiment could have tolerated a 'confused and disgusting' administration to have existed for a day.

They concluded in other words, that the Governor and the Regimental Commander were beyond criticism; anyone who criticized them, their administration or institutions, was necessarily guilty of 'extraordinary conduct'.

The interesting aspect of this petty deception is that not one of the officers dared to cast a slur on Barry's reputation as a doctor. Her professional integrity was unquestioned even among her enemies.

Barry was not deterred by the Board's finding. She did not doubt the justice of her claim for a moment. When she was ordered to the West Indies the following November she asked the Colonial Office to refund the money to a friend, a Mr Thomas Powett Hayes, who would give a receipt for it on her account.

Even when she was abroad, Barry worried at the Government for an answer. She argued that the Governor had recognized her claim for civil pay when she first arrived on the island; that recognition in her view could not be invalidated by the report of a Board of Medical Officers 'adverse to me and my measures for the benefit of the poor coloured part of the community'. The Governor himself and the Military Chaplain, neither of them friends of hers, had admitted, even complained, that the sick poor of the island suffered after her departure. Be that as it may, her claim was shelved. The Health Officer, a Mr Reed, a former Assistant Surgeon to the East India Company, was appointed to her old post in December 1837. This gentleman preferred inspecting the ships to caring for the poor, and he made it a lucrative job. In addition to his salary of 10s. a day he charged 10s. 6d. a day for his advice to seamen and 21s. to the Captain and passengers, plus extra for medicine. His other duties plainly went by the board. Mr McClaren, the Assistant Surgeon of the civil hospital, remarked in 1838 that the sick poor were totally neglected. Mr Reed had refused to visit them and some had died because of the neglect. As Barry would have said, no comment is necessary.

9

Sworn to Secrecy

Barry left England for the West Indies six months after she had been sent home in disgrace. Her name was cleared. No official action was taken against her, yet she was demoted from Principal Medical Officer to Staff Surgeon and it seems clear, reading between the lines, that the posting to the Windward and Leeward Islands was designed to settle her in a station where her reforming zeal would not involve political complications.

Once again she was to serve in one of the most unhealthy outposts of the Empire. The voyage proved a dispiriting experience for her: 'cabined, cribbed, confined' for weeks on end, she had to exist on a diet of stale biscuits, rancid butter and tainted water. She drank coffee (the only stimulant she now permitted herself) without milk and craved for fresh fruit and vegetables.

The days and nights were monotonous and the flapping of the sails in the wind and the creaking of the ship's masts frayed her nerves. But she knew that, compared to the troops huddled below in semi-darkness with a bare eighteen inches between their swaying hammocks, her quarters were comfort itself. The stench below was dreadful. The soldiers suffered from lack of fresh air, fresh food and any proper sanitation. The result was that the ships-at-war had a terrible death rate. Morale, too, was low on the journey out, for the troops were filled with foreboding. By now the West Indies had gained an awesome reputation in the service. 'The Cradle of Fever' was the popular name given to the Windward and Leeward Islands.

British Guiana on the mainland, which was a part of the station, was nicknamed 'The Abode of Death'.

Parliament itself was alarmed at the rate of sickness and death among the troops in the West Indies. Between 1816 and 1848 only ten of the forty regiments stationed in the Windward and Leeward Islands escaped yellow fever or 'black vomit', as it was graphically called. And other diseases threatened the troops too: malaria, 'inflammation of the lungs' – twice as deadly as in Great Britain – and chronic dysentery, from which one in five of the sufferers died.

After the commotion she had caused in St Helena and her court-martial, it seems unlikely that the posting to such a formidable area was accidental, though of course Barry did enjoy an uncomfortable respect at headquarters for her interest in the troops' welfare (the service in those days was small and every individual officer was personally known to the Army Medical Department). In March 1839, shortly after Dr Barry landed on the island of Antigua, Sir Andrew Halliday, Deputy Inspector General of Army Hospitals, wrote an open letter to the Secretary at War, Lord Howick, emphasizing that 'much of the sickness and not a little of the mortality of the troops was caused by the indifference towards the comfort and conveniences of the soldier and to the total disregard of all means of prevention'.

Pernickety, bad-tempered, frail and fastidious – one could call Barry all those things, and ludicrous as well. Yet this small and curious person raised the standards of medicine and touched the public conscience about the condition of the most degraded members of society – the prisoners, the paupers, the blacks and the lunatics – wherever she went.

It can hardly be coincidental that the year she arrived the Governor of Antigua urged the local government to abandon 'the objectionable practice which prevails in these islands of detaining lunatics in prison' and called for a 'report on the conditions of the lunatics from the Medical Officer'. By March 1840, mad men and women formerly confined in 'dark and ill-ventilated cellars so injurious to their bodily health and mental restoration' were transferred to the military hospital.

Another echo of Barry's insistence on high medical standards is reflected in the Governor of Antigua's proclamation in 1840 prohibiting unqualified persons from 'practising physic and vending medicines either as physician, surgeon or apothecary...'

She was by now a middle-aged woman in her forties, an elderly woman by the standards of those day. Yet she had heavy responsibilities which involved a good deal of travel in the stifling heat. Barbados, Trinidad, Tobago, Grenada, St Vincent's and St Lucia, Dominica, Antigua with Monserrat, St Kitt's with Scotia and British Guiana on the mainland were all part of the Windward and Leeward Islands. As a doctor, Barry was constantly called from station to station – there was rarely a regiment without an epidemic. Steamships now plied between the islands and at least saved her from some of the discomforts of travelling under canvas.

She carried her little dog aboard in her arms, insisted on her own cabin, and liked to have the goat which supplied her with fresh milk comfortably quartered too! Her sword, it was said, was as long as herself and she always took an umbrella on her journeys. In the service she was becoming something of a legend.

One senses that by the time she had settled in the West Indies, Barry had at last accepted her lonely and ambiguous role in life. In the autumn of 1840, when the retiring Inspector General of Hospitals went home to England, and before his replacement arrived, Barry acted as temporary Medical Director, in charge of the health of the troops in the command. Evidently she not only did useful work but also received public acknowledgement for it; she was thanked in General Orders for her conduct of the Department. By 1842, she was once again appointed Principal Medical Officer, this time in Trinidad. She settled in a country house 'a gunshot from St James's Barracks about two miles from Port of Spain'. She seems to have been a highly respected officer, often seen at Government levées.

But she had not mellowed altogether. When a fellow officer, Dr Bradford, described her in an official report as 'about 50', she flew into a rage and accused him of a 'dastardly attempt to blast my fair prospects'. (She was in fact forty-three.) For all her brilliant reputation, Barry was still insecure – which, with her secret and her past, was hardly surprising.

All her life she showed not only compassion, but a vivid ability to sympathize with the individual sufferer and her reports on disease stand out from the dry, abstract remarks and erudite phraseology of her colleagues. Her answers to a circular sent to Medical Officers asking them about the cause, symptom and treatment of *delirium tremens* – a common complaint amongst the troops – are written almost journalistically, quoting the individual sufferer. 'It is almost impossible to end the habit' (of heavy drinking), she wrote, 'where to use the patient's own words, "the weather is always so hot, rum always so cheap and a man always so dry"; the only chance would be to embark that subject in a Temperance vessel with plenty of nutritious diet.'

She had no doubt that the 'continued use and abuse of ardent spirits' was the root cause of *delirium tremens* and described the onset of the illness as 'ferocious delirium', which gave place to trembling nervous delirium: 'every species of blue devils torment the sufferer inducing him, if not watched often, to commit suicide . . .' Treatment, she recommended, should vary according to the patient. It included 'stimuli such as brandy, champaign, pepiscum, etc., keeping the bowels open and a light diet'. These were occasionally helpful in the first and second attacks; beyond that there was little one could do.

Since Barry herself was a teetotaller, the report reveals her detachment and also shows how closely she had observed the life of the ordinary soldier.

As a doctor, she recognized the need for order and cleanliness in the wards but her patients liked her and trusted her skill. She could be a martinet one minute, snapping at a forgetful orderly who had not carried out her instructions to the letter, and infinitely kind and gentle with a suffering soldier the next. Once, when she noticed an orderly struggling to write a letter for a dying patient, she offered to help him acquire an education. By now she had become a true Victorian – pious, keen on self-improvement and something of a moralist.

She made an extraordinary impression on all who met her that lasted for years. An observer who signed himself 'Captain', wrote to the *Lancet* thirty years after Barry's death, giving a detailed account of their meeting.

It was in the year 1844 that I was sent from Barbados to Trinidad to sit on a general court martial . . . On the assembling of court, an individual appeared as spectator who at once attracted my attention. He was in the full dress of an army surgeon but had all the appearance of being a woman . . . I was told that the individual was Dr Barry, the principal medical officer of the district. The impression and general belief was that he was a hermaphrodite and as such escaped much comment or observation in places where everyone was used to him . . . But I was convinced James Barry was a woman about 60 years of age [*she was only 45!*] *and being much interested in him, I cultivated his acquaintance and became very friendly. He frequently asked me to visit him and I endeavoured to draw out his antecedents, but found him very reticent.*

No wonder Barry was regarded as tetchy and difficult by her colleagues. She must have sensed that behind their apparent friendliness lay a desire to fathom her mystery. To remain aloof must have been a strain to a nature with so much generosity in it, but she could never allow herself the pleasure of normal human relationships.

Another correspondent who served with her in Trinidad also retained a vivid impression of her. A month after her death in 1865, he wrote to a local paper in Cumberland for details 'of that extraordinary person ... always suspected of being a female from his effeminate features and voice and having neither beard nor whiskers'. Dr Barry was 'a very bold person and challenged one or two of our officials for naming him a diminutive creature ... it was currently said that he had made a will leaving the dog all his effects and "Sambo" his black servant a legacy of £100'.

Barry had seen so much death on the islands that it is hardly surprising that she should have made a will. She obviously realized that despite her care in personal hygiene and the precautions she took against infection, she was at risk every time she tended a patient. Sir Andrew Halliday, Deputy-Inspector General of Hospitals, had recommended that no troops should remain in a Colony for more than two years. Barry had been stationed in Trinidad for almost three years, and had served in the West Indies as a whole for six.

In 1845 she at last succumbed to yellow fever. For the first time in thirty-two years' service she was herself a patient. She gave instructions to Dr O'Connor, the doctor attending her, and to the lady of the house (a friend of hers) that if she died her body should be rolled up in the sheets and buried in her nightshirt without an examination. She faced up to death coolly, with a minimum of fuss.

But her illness caused anxiety among the junior officers – and perhaps curiosity. A tale was told at a regimental dinner in 1881 to a Colonel Rogers, by a fellow officer 'who had never mentioned the subject before'.

I was quartered as a subaltern in Trinidad while Dr Barry was serving there in the capacity of Principal Medical Officer. One day a friend of mine, the Assistant Surgeon, asked me to walk with him into Port of Spain. 'The P.M.O.' said he 'is down with fever at the house of a lady-friend, but has given a strict injunction to us not to visit him. Nevertheless, I feel bound to call and see how he is, will you come with me?' On arrival my friend entered Barry's bed-room, while I remained on the verandah smoking a cheroot. He called me excitedly into the room, exclaiming as he flung back the bed-clothes, 'See Barry is a woman!'

At that moment the P.M.O. awoke to consciousness and gazed at us bewilderingly. But she quickly recovered presence of mind and asked us, in low tones, to swear solemnly not to disclose her secret as long as she lived.

The slight flaw in this story is that Colonel Rogers had published a novel in 1881, *A Modern Sphinx*, about Barry and was anxious to whip up interest in the subject. In the concluding paragraph of his letter to the *Lancet*, written from the Savage Club, Rogers added: 'In view of the great interest revived by this correspondence, I shall without delay bring out a cheap edition of my novel *A Modern Sphinx*.'

Despite the romantic flavour of Rogers' account, another letter from an officer who served in Trinidad at the time corroborates the incident. Forty years later, Colonel T. de Montmorency recalled his experience:

I was not actually in the room when Dr James Barry's sex was discovered in 1841 [1845 actually, but a forgivable error at a distance of forty years]; the matter was confidentially told to me immediately after the discovery by one of the party present, so I would not wish that either his name, nor mine, be brought before the public in this matter.

There is too much evidence here to sweep away – and yet not quite enough to be conclusive. Perhaps it was as well, with such a scandal simmering below the surface, that Dr Barry should go home to England. She arrived on Boxing Day, 1845. 'Home, sick', she writes laconically in her record of service and she stayed at home on leave until November 1846.

10

The Soldier's Disease

'Never in better health or more jolly', wrote Assistant Surgeon George Lawson, one of Barry's fellow officers, breaking his journey to the Crimea at Malta. Sir Walter Scott described its capital, Valetta (where Barry was to spend her next five years), as 'a dream' and other writers admired the island too. Coleridge enjoyed his stay as Private Secretary to the Civil Commissioner and Thackeray, on a P. & O. cruise, wrote a racy description for a travel book. Malta, in those days, consisted of steep streets with steps all the way up and houses on either side. Tinkers, tailors and shoemakers sat outside their front doors working. For educated nineteenth-century travellers Malta, with its noble architecture of soft, golden stone, its palms, hibiscus and archaeological treasures, was a magnificent, magical island.

Barry arrived there late in November 1846. After her long stint in the tropics and almost a year spent at home recuperating from her severe attack of yellow fever, she was, it seemed, at last to serve in a pleasant post. She was once again appointed Principal Medical Officer of the station with imposing quarters in keeping with her position. For Dr Barry, however, it was not only the lofty houses of white stone that impressed, but also the stench from the sewers that wafted up even to the most elegant drawing-rooms. For Malta was an island of tourists' delights – and disease.

The island, like many of the stations in which Barry served, was extremely unhealthy. The death rate in 1851 was more than one in fifty in the towns, and one in thirty-five in the villages – more than twice the death rate in Great Britain.

Barry was nearly fifty. She had spent twenty-two years in the Army Medical Department. By now she was a very experienced physician who, through her clinical work, her careful observation of disease and her constant study of contemporary medical literature kept up-to-date with the latest developments in science. However, like the rest of her generation, she was ignorant of the true cause of cholera. She believed that it was 'miasma', foul vapours from matter polluted by excrement or refuse of any kind, that in itself caused infection. This theory that breathing in evil air brought on such diseases as cholera and typhus was widely accepted by Victorian medical men. It was not until thirty-five years later that Robert Koch, the brilliant German scientist, isolated and identified the cholera bacillus.

But if the causes were unknown at the time, the effects – violent diarrhoea, dehydration and frequently death – were all too well known. Cholera had ravaged Malta ten years earlier. Panic spread among the people at that time. Mothers refused to go near their children, husbands their wives, and in a family of eight brothers, not one had the courage to go near his father's death bed. And these were people in the educated upper classes, not peasants. People even hinted that the doctors themselves had refused to treat cholera patients.

Within a year of her posting as Principal Medical Officer on the island, a mysterious disease broke out and the newspapers began to report the suspicion of the 'awful visitation of Cholera'. One writer even solemnly suggested banning the pigeons from ships in quarantine from flying into the harbour.

Barry had treated cholera in different parts of the world and we need not doubt her reaction to the rumours of a fresh outbreak even though cholera could kill within hours as did some of the drastic 'cures' of the day, electric shocks and boiling baths.

The Governor of the island was 'desirous' that Dr Barry should examine some civilian patients in a village where an outbreak of cholera was feared. So in mid-September 1848, accompanied by a police physician, a Dr Collings attached to the Palace, and two other military medical officers, Barry went to the Casal, a marshy coastal village near Valetta.

When the party arrived on the spot, a policeman approached

and whispered some word to Dr Collings, who apparently in an ecstasy, turned to Barry crying, 'Aha, Dr Barry, you cannot now crow over us, here are two cases of Cholera.'

'I was shocked and disgusted at this unChristian burst of indecent joy – these expressions need no explanation and on them I shall make no comment,' she reported to the Governor. 'We proceeded to examine this poor woman.' All the doctors declared that the disease was not Cholera . . . 'Nothing could exceed [her] misery and destitution – without covering, or food and in the act of sucking a piece of orange.' The village physician told the doctors that he had given her calomel and opium. 'The effort was made to restore her but she perished.'

Professional jealousy, which Barry often aroused, is revealed in Dr Collings's outburst. What also emerges from her report is that after more than thirty years of seeing wretched poverty and disease, she was still personally concerned with every case.

The doctors made 'minute inspection' of the corpse and could only suppose that the woman had been a victim of 'Sporadic Cholera', which Barry described as a severe affection of the stomach and bowels and prevalent in all countries at certain seasons. She believed that the dead patient had 'only required nourishment and attention to be restored to health'. The local doctor was convinced that the cause of death was typhus fever. The fact was that given the level of medical knowledge at the time, none of them was in a position to make an accurate diagnosis.

Next the medical team visited 'a poor man with a large family'. He too was in a state of miserable poverty: 'We were fortunate enough to obtain for him, what he most needed – sustenance – and he eventually recovered for I saw him afterwards.' They unanimously agreed that his illness was not cholera.

They finally saw the two other cases.

A boy about twelve years of age stretched on a handful of straw on the ground in an open yard under stone stairs, affected with well marked and not to be mistaken Typhus Fever; in an adjoining hovel, an old woman quite as scantily provided for in the last states of Fever of a very malignant Typhoid Type. These wretched beings were in the most deplorable plight, surrounded by filth and stench intolerable, without sustenance or support. In fact, I feel inadequate to describe the scene and shrunk from it with horror.

But she did speak to the local doctor and discovered that the villagers of Casal suffered from remittant and typhus fever every year, owing to the marshy, badly drained land, as well as 'their being miserably poor and crowded'.

With her usual commonsense, Barry showed concern about the open sewers around Valetta which polluted the atmosphere, particularly near the pig sties. They brought on disease 'equally destructive, if not more so, than the so much dreaded Cholera', she said. (Although she did not realize it, the open sewers were an indirect cause of cholera, not because of the stench they gave off, but because drinking polluted water from wells near open sewers or from contaminated rivers was the most common way of contracting the disease.)

In medical matters she remained cool and logical, although she reacted indignantly to unnecessary suffering. She closed this letter, written in October 1848, to the Assistant Military Secretary, Major Pipson, on a note which must have seemed off-key to the sporting, military set.

'However, should it please almighty God to inflict this awful scourge on us, we have only to commit ourselves to the never failing mercies of Our Heavenly Father and with deep humility and resignation, bowing down to say "O Lord, Thy will be done".'

As she grew older, no doubt as a result of the life she had lived and the suffering she had seen, Barry became increasingly and explicitly religious. From her earliest days at the Cape, she had worked actively to ensure that even the most abject members of society – the lepers and the paupers – should not lack the consolation of religion. Nowhere in her writings did she suggest that religion should be used to reconcile wretched human beings to their condition. On the contrary, her blazing humanism contrasted with those Evangelists who, in their passion to save souls, persuaded their converts that suffering in this life was a preparation for triumph in the next. Implicit in all her attitudes is a rebellion against a social order which reduced people to squalor.

By upbringing a Roman Catholic, yet compelled to conform to the established church for the sake of her career, Barry was forced into a position of religious tolerance remarkable for her time; in her eyes the spirit of the thing was always more important than the outward show. For most of the officers attending Church Parade on Sunday was merely a matter of form, an automatic display of piety. For Barry, however, her devotions obviously helped her to come to terms with the misery she witnessed during her routine work.

As the epidemic spread, the troops themselves were affected. On the 6th of October Barry sent in a report on the death and post-mortem of a soldier in the Artillery. She found herself at odds with a Dr Richardson who maintained that the cause of death was Asiatic cholera and not sporadic cholera as she believed. This disagreement displeased the Governor who wanted his medical officers to present a united front. He demanded an explanation of the difference between the two diseases. Barry explained that it was 'very minute', and she proceeded to outline, in a highly technical manner, the medical distinction between them. In her exposition she quoted the work of a young doctor, Dr E. A. Parkes, an Assistant Physician at University College, who held the very advanced theory that cholera caused chemical changes in the blood.

However the Governor had no time for scientific niceties. He believed that medical officers should 'find some grounds for agreement, both as regards the credit of the Profession and the safety of the Public'. But his wish for doctors to sink their disagreements in order to present a show of unity, was one that no honest, openminded intellectual could accept.

'With the greatest deference and respect', she begged to be excused from agreeing with His Excellency's views. She added:

> It is proverbial that all professions, whether legal, ecclesiastical or medical differ and seldom arrive at the same conclusion as to the cause and effect of things; in fact the world in general disagrees . . . I even presume to contend that such equality of opinion would in no wise add to the credit of the Profession or ensure the safety of the Public.

Here she was astute enough to appeal to the Governor to review his own experience. 'Perhaps cases have come under His Excellency's notice even among his own friends, where one physician differing in opinion from the other has had the most beneficial effects.'

She instanced three cases from her own professional life when she had disagreed with other doctors about the patients' treatment 'where it has pleased the Almighty in his divine providence to make me the humble instrument of their recovery'! She referred to her most recent success – saving the life of a sea captain's daughter in Malta – by adopting different measures from the doctors previously employed on the case and in particular to the time when Lord Charles Somerset lay dangerously ill. If the Governor wanted corroboration, she suggested that he should refer to Fitzroy Somerset, the Military Secretary.

The Governor, of course, would have preferred more simple and expedient explanations for complex problems. But Barry's intellectual honesty would not allow her to pander to this preference. Where medicine was concerned she was not arrogant. She went out of her way to emphasize that her experience was not unique: 'perhaps there are few Medical Officers of any experience who cannot quote parallel instances'.

But she did deplore the military medical officers' indiscretion in allowing the troops to get wind of the fact that cholera was suspected. 'Giving publicity to anything that might excite panic among the troops . . . could only drive them to despair, drunkenness and death: every Soldier looking on a case of Cholera as a Forlorn Hope.'

Sanitary conditions on Malta were appalling and Barry knew it. Barracks and military hospitals were overcrowded, dark and stuffy. The latrines were foul, the water supply from the open tanks polluted. She evidently had endless interviews with the Governor on the subject. 'I shall always feel happy in expressing my acknowledgement for His Excellency's kindness and courtesy on those occasions, and I feel proud to add His Excellency not infrequently condescended to approve of measures suggested by me.'

Ten years earlier her biting comments on the 'confused and disgusting' state of the hospitals at St Helena had resulted in a court-martial and caused her to be sent home under arrest. But in maturity, she had grown wiser in handling those in high office although she was still resolute when a matter of principle was involved. Only her methods of maintaining her standards had changed – she had learned that tact was often the most efficient way of handling superiors.

The exact cause of the mysterious outbreak of illness in 1848 was never discovered. Although a great part of the island's population contracted the disease, only sixteen died – a tribute, perhaps, to the energy and commonsense of Barry and her colleagues.

Not until the Crimean War brought home to the British public the widespread suffering of thousands of British troops, due to insanitary conditions, did the authorities recognize that public health was important as Barry had always known it to be. Only then were the conditions of barracks and hospitals improved on a wide scale. Her protest alone could never wrest more than limited reforms from the innately conservative and tight-fisted military establishment.

They did recognize her work, however. She records in a memorandum that she received 'the thanks of the Duke of Wellington for my services during the period that Island was visited by the cholera'.

From Malta she sailed directly to her next post in the Mediterranean, the island of Corfu.

11

A Tittle-Tattle Place

In Corfu Dr Barry gained her first promotion for twenty-four years. She was upgraded to Deputy Inspector General, bypassing the ranks of Assistant Inspector and Brevet Deputy Inspector. The affair of the court-martial had been blotted out by her good work in the West Indies and Malta. At her new rank she was an officer of considerable importance. Had she been a typical British officer, instead of an oddity, she would have thoroughly enjoyed the life of the island.

For Corfu had an umistakably 'English' quality. The officers played cricket at the Byron Cricket Club; swaggered along the Esplanade with its palms, cypresses and orange trees; or galloped, red coats flying, in chase across the island. And their ladies enjoyed themselves too at the endless balls, dinner parties and picnics. The military families of officer class lived in lordly style, in gabled and balconied Venetian buildings; a house with a bathroom was known as an 'English house'.

When Barry arrived in April 1851 (she went straight from Malta without taking home leave) the weather was perfect. From her window she had a magnificent view of mountains and limpid blue sea, and for once she was serving on a pleasant and healthy station where no fearful disease ravaged the troops or the population.

However, there were certain disadvantages. Edward Lear, who was on the island during Barry's sojourn, thought Corfu a 'very small tittle-tattle place'. What mattered to the fashionable military men and their wives was the turnout of the troops, the drilling, the salutes and the parades. Barry, although a stickler for discipline in hospital, where it could affect the treatment of her patients, objected to this empty exercise. She tried vainly to stop commanders drilling their men in the midday sun and filling her hospitals with sunstroke cases. Even on the hottest days she could be seen straggling along on a tall, lean horse, an orderly on either side, seeking with shrill insistence to dissuade the officers from this ritual. The 'interfering ways' of the tiny, eccentric Medical Officer were resented by the Colonels and Commanders who were very grand personages in their own esteem. But, as a member of the troops, tended by her when 'quite a lad', wrote to *Lloyd's Weekly Newspaper* forty-five years later, 'there must be many officers, and a great many of the rank and file, who remember her with gratitude'.

One gentleman who certainly did not retain grateful memories of her was Colonel Denny, Commander of the 71st Highland Light Infantry. At two o'clock one afternoon, in the full glare of the sun, the Colonel was leading his regiment over the draw-bridge to drill them on the Esplanade (where, no doubt, the ladies with their parasols would be watching) when Barry, flourishing a horse-whip, halted him. In front of his troops she threatened to report him for his folly. Whether by accident or not, Barry's horse-whip caught the splendid-looking officer full in the face. Infuriated, he grabbed her whip and flung it into the moat, and was just about to send her after it when a friendly bystander intervened. According to the story, she convened a medical board and declared the gallant Colonel to be *'non compos mentis'*.

As she aged, the two distinct sides of her character grew more marked: the passionate termagant, shrilling at authority and making enemies everywhere, and the infinitely generous and patient doctor. She was 'punctuality itself', frightened the orderlies by her scathing comments if she detected a 'stench' and demanded that military officers at the hospital should be in uniform to meet her. And when patients assembled at the clinic for her inspection she walked up and down the rows muttering 'Dirty beasts, dirty beasts, go home and wash yourselves!' But the soldiers also remembered her regularly giving a dollar to a private who delivered a few choice oranges from her own private supply (brought especially by mail steamer from

Naples and Sicily) to needy patients in the wards. 'To the sick', wrote an orderly who had served with her, Dr Barry was the 'most kind and humane gentleman ever met, but patients who contracted disease through their own folly – and these were not a few – he would not look at'.

In May 1852 she returned to England on her first home leave for six years.

Barry was no longer young, and she had spent many testing and difficult years abroad: she was impatient, bad-tempered and very, very vulnerable. In London society she was generally considered to be a woman, and her hostesses usually warned their friends of her extraordinary appearance and eccentric behaviour before she arrived. Wherever she went, Psyche, her little poodle, and a black servant accompanied her.

For a time she lived in Down Street, Piccadilly. She was frequently seen about in the company of Lady Charles Somerset, the widow of her dear friend. Perhaps the two women drew consolation from each other's company and from memories of those golden days at the Cape.

Another member of the Beaufort family who watched her progress kindly was the first Fitzroy Somerset, Lord Charles's youngest brother, now Lord Raglan. In October 1852, during Barry's home leave, he had been elevated to the peerage, on the death of the Duke of Wellington. Having served the Duke loyally and bravely in the Peninsular War, and as Military Secretary at the Horse Guards for twenty-five years, he had hoped to become Commander-in-Chief of the Army himself but to his disappointment Lord Hardinge had been preferred. As a consolation Fitzroy Somerset was offered a peerage. Queen Victoria herself was willing to 'bear the cost of the fees' of his investiture, since he displayed some reluctance to accept, and in the circumstances he could hardly refuse.

Was Dr Barry, always such a close friend of the family, present at the ceremony? Certainly Lord Raglan – as Fitzroy Somerset became – thought highly enough of her to send a note of introduction to the British Ambassador in Vienna when she passed through on her way back to Corfu. It contained the usual excuses for her eccentricity, and the commendation that she had given excellent service, particularly in South Africa.

Through this introduction perhaps she was asked to give professional aid to a crew member of Archduke Maximilian's staff. Evidently the treatment was successful, for through the British Government in Corfu Barry received tangible recognition of His Imperial Highness's gratitude in the form of a magnificent diamond ring.

When she reported back for duty in Corfu in March 1853 war with Russia was already imminent. The Tsar, eager to expand his power by taking Constantinople and thus gaining dominance in the Mediterranean, was looking for a quarrel with Turkey. He found it in a dispute over the custody of the Holy Places in Jerusalem, then a part of the Turkish Empire, policed by Turkish Mohammedans. The Tsar's Greek Orthodox monks, egged on by Tsar Nicholas, refused to allow the Roman Catholic monks, supported by the French, to place a silver star over the manger at Bethlehem or to keep the golden key to the church. The quarrel grew bitter and riots and killings of some Orthodox monks followed. The Tsar immediately blamed the Turkish police and marched towards the Danube on a crusade to protect the Orthodox Christian subjects from Islam. The British saw the Russian expansion as a threat to their naval power. When the Russian Black Sea fleet caught the Turkish navy off the south shore of the Black Sea at Sinope, and sank every ship, the British howled with rage at the 'massacre'! Honour required Britannia to declare war in defence of Turkish independence and an expeditionary force was dispatched to the Crimea.

On the 27th of March Queen Victoria's Message of War was read out in the Commons. A wave of patriotism surged throughout the country. As the first battalions of Guards marched, with drums beating, towards the troopships, cheering crowds lined the streets. However, very few of the 30 000 men who sailed for Turkey had the remotest idea what they were fighting for.

As soon as Barry heard that war had broken out, she volunteered for a posting to the battle front. She was told that there was no vacancy for an officer of her rank. Never one to give up easily, she then suggested to Lord Raglan and Dr John Hall, Inspector General of Hospitals, that the sick and wounded 'packed into hospital tents to make room for the new arrivals, pale, dirty and shivering' should be sent to Corfu to be nursed back to health. Dr John Hall, later honoured for his services in the war, was described by Florence Nightingale as 'Knight of the Crimean Burial Grounds'. Cholera, dysentery, starvation and above all lack of military planning were decimating the Army.

By the late autumn of 1854, nearly a quarter of the troops were dying. Lord Raglan, desperately trying to cope, was angered by *The Times*'s attack on the lethargy of the army besieging Sebastopol and on the incompetence of its commanders. For the first time people at home were learning the truth about the living conditions of British soldiers serving abroad.

On the 27th of January 1855 Dr Hall noted in his diary that Lord Raglan's temper was 'at boiling point' because of all the criticism of the medical services and added: 'I would be glad to get away, though I am conscious of having exerted myself to my utmost ability . . . it is possible that his Lordship wants to get rid of me and make room for his protégé Barry . . . if so well and good – but don't persecute other people.'

One could find reasons, of course, why a gentlemanly gentleman like Lord Raglan, conventional to the core, might not entirely welcome his protégé Barry in the Crimea. He did, however, accept her suggestion to ship the sick and wounded troops to Corfu.

On the 17th of February the transport *Dunbar* brought 462 of the wretched men – sick and ragged, verminous and neglected – into port. They were suffering from cholera, fever, bullet wounds and frostbite.

The order and cleanliness in Barry's hospital in Corfu must have seemed like heaven to them. By the end of the month, she had fifty-three of the Crimean veterans fit for duty again. Sixty-three were well enough for 'slight duty', sixty-nine were patients in bed, and 260 attending the hospital for treatment. Only seventeen of Dr Barry's patients died, which, considering that in Scutari during the same period men were perishing at the rate of twenty-three a day, was a creditable result.

As always, her concern for her patients brought Barry into conflict with her superiors. The arrival of the sick and wounded created problems for the complacent military authorities; they were more worried about money than men. They had to decide on rates of pay for the invalids and provide new uniforms for the troops who had arrived in rags 'infested to such a degree with vermin' that they had to be destroyed. They also had to find accommodation for the invalids. By April there was not a house or a public building vacant. The island seemed to be overrun with sick and convalescent troops, with the result that the social life of the military élite suffered. Before long it became difficult 'to induce the officers to stay on an island where there is no society, no shooting and no amusements of any kind'.

Major-General MacIntosh, G.O.C. of the Ionian Islands, was keen to ship the post-convalescent soldiers back to the war. On the 1st of April he inspected 213 of the men passed as fit for duty by Dr Barry, and embarked them on board two troopships bound for Turkey (H.M.S. *Sidon* and H.M.S. *Leopard*). The ships were already packed and only ninety-three of the men could be taken back to the Crimea. Consequently, the G.O.C. was left with 120 troops passed as fit, but 'with no arms or accoutrements' for their usual duties. They were put on fatigue. This infuriated Deputy Inspector General James Barry. She wanted her ex-patients to rest during the sea voyage before they returned to battle. Instead, they were to be given pointless tasks in the hot sun. Barry warned the C.O. to desist and threatened to report the whole affair to Lord Raglan.

General MacIntosh was uneasy. He did not believe that Barry had the influence she boasted of and yet he did not feel he could entirely ignore the affair. He sent a report to Lord Raglan saying that 'Dr Barry had tried to impress Methuen (the men's Commanding Officer) by stating that he was a private friend of yours and had resided 13 years in the house of your Lordship's brother'.

Further the General objected to Barry's 'injudicious interference with the management of the men' after they had been pronounced fit, but was anxious to 'apprehend his, Barry's, having endeavoured to give erroneous impressions as to the treatment they have received ... Should Dr Barry have written to Lord Raglan', he concluded, 'I feel quite convinced that your Lordship's mind will in no manner be biased ...'

Lord Raglan replied with the tact for which he was well known:

I am sorry to learn that Dr Barry, of whose zeal for the service I entertain no doubt, should have thought fit to interfere in a matter . . . which rested with you alone. You will be glad to learn that he has not written to me and I should hope that he may, upon reflection, feel that such a course would not only be improper, but would be utterly disapproved by me.

On June 28th 1855, not long after that letter was written, Lord Raglan died. Officially the cause of death was attributed to 'Crimean fever'. One of his soldiers described him as a 'dear old Christian Gentleman who had died of a broken heart'. He had seen the British Army that he had loved and worked for all his life, starved and frozen to death in the winter of 1854. His tragedy was that he never recognized the extent of his own incompetence. He had fought gallantly at Wellington's side in the Peninsular War and had lost his right arm at the Battle of Waterloo, but since then he had never been near a battlefield. And for a quarter of a century he had been bound to his desk at the Horse Guards. At sixty-seven he was simply not fit to take command. With his death, Barry lost her last link with the Beauforts.

Nevertheless, she had made plans to visit the Crimea during her leave. No record appears to exist of what Barry actually did there. In her account she confines herself to the comment that she had spent three months with the 4th Division before Sebastopol 'and made myself useful as opportunities offered'. Before she even arrived the news that Dr Barry was planning to visit the Crimea spread like wildfire among the Medical Officers.

'I had a letter from Corfu announcing that Dr Barry had left on a pleasure trip to the Crimea, accompanied by his horse, his goat, his dogs and servants', wrote Dr Linton from Scutari. 'He paid us a visit in passing . . . but he did not honour us with the company of any of the animals . . .'

And an even more acid warning arrived from Hall's second-in-command, Dr Cummings.

I may as well warn you that you are to have a visit from the renowned Dr Barry. He called on me yesterday and as I never met him before, his appearance and conversation rather surprised me. He appears to be in his dotage and is an intolerable bore, so I would recommend you to be prepared for him as he seems to have the intention of quartering himself on you. He has with him his horse and his servant. He will expect you to listen to every quarrel he has had since coming into the service . . . You probably know they are not a few.

Barry was obviously disliked, and even feared by her colleagues. She had kept herself aloof from them for obvious reasons and irritated them by the passion with which she threw herself into her work. As a result medical colleagues tended to talk and write about her in tones of malice. Dr Linton, who never actually saw the servants and animals, added a goat to the dog and the servant which Dr Cummings mentioned.

By this time Florence Nightingale and her devoted supporters were beginning to introduce some order into the chaos of Crimean hospitals. Not surprisingly the Army Medical Department was becoming increasingly sensitive to criticism. It had proved hopelessly inadequate during the winter of 1854, and was still badly organized and inefficient, lacking in men, supplies and the ability to improvise. *The Times* reporter, William Howard Russell, brought home the miseries of the men in the trenches to an indignant public. In the autumn of 1855 one of Florence Nightingale's supporters, Mrs Bracebridge, delivered a lecture in Coventry, attacking the surgeons for ignorance and callousness and describing the shocking state of the hospitals. Mrs Bracebridge gave her shocked audience specific, but inaccurate, examples of doctors ill-treating the troops.

In the face of this onslaught, Barry remained loyal to her Department. When Sir John Hall approached her for her comments on his counter-attack to the Sanitary Commission's critical report on the hospitals in the Crimea, she somewhat surprisingly supported him, although she herself had never tolerated dirt, or inadequate provisions.

Many thanks for your 'Observations' which I read with deep interest – the Dept has been treated in a most extraordinary manner. How is it that Dr Sutherland was placed on this last commission which I humbly opine will be worse than nothing? . . . How is it that you are not on the Royal Commission? I hear they are going to send a lot of Medical officers to India. Will the Commissioners and Civilians be despatched also? – they shd all go in the same boat. Pray say all manner of kind things for me to Lady Hall. I should have liked to have seen your young ones especially the little Lord Chancellor if you had been in London.

Plainly Barry felt that civilians were outsiders who could not possibly understand the background to the disastrous muddle. And when Barry met Florence Nightingale, the Deputy Inspector General did not hesitate to show her displeasure. Miss Nightingale wrote of the encounter, which must have rankled for years, after Barry's death.

I never had such a blackguard rating in my life – I who have had more than any woman – than from Barry sitting on [her] horse while I was crossing the hospital square with only my cap on in the sun. [She] kept me standing in the midst of a crowd of soldiers, commissariats, servants, camp followers, etc., everyone of whom behaved like a gentleman during the scolding I received while [she] behaved like a brute. After she was dead I was told she was a woman. I should say she was the most hardened creature I ever met throughout the army.

These two, perhaps the most remarkable women in Britain, were destined to quarrel – the withered little General, who had worked her way up in a man's world with a man's methods, and the ruthless reformer who used feminine wiles and feminine bullying to get her own way. 'A woman', wrote Miss Nightingale, 'obtains that from military courtesy . . . which a man . . . partly from temper, partly from policy is effectually banned.'

While other officers did not dare to criticize openly a civilian and a female who threatened their authority, Barry felt no such compunction. She stood in no awe of a woman who could organize, who could reform. She may well have wondered what all the fuss was about.

Back in Corfu, she kept herself busy as usual. When she returned, Colonel Lockyear of the 97th Regiment wrote to her from Malta, where nearly 100 men were suffering from cholera:

he had neither medicines nor medical comforts for his troops who had just been ordered to Piraeus and no means of obtaining them. 'Within two hours of getting the letter', Barry wrote, 'I had embarked a supply of comforts and medicines for the use of the Regiment and Hospital' – and she continued to send supplies once a week, since there was no other way of getting them through. She also sent similar help to the Commanding Officers of the 3rd Buffs and of the 91st Regiments and the Director General of the Army Medical Department, as well as the Commanding Officers, thanked her for her help.

Poor Barry. There was no one to report her story, no one to acclaim her. She herself had to remind the authorities, in a memorandum at the end of her life, of her service 'in a career which impartially may be deemed to have been useful and faithful one'.

12

Changes and Chances

'No-one can feel about the army as I do', wrote Florence Nightingale in a private note in February 1857. The heroine of the Crimean War, the darling of the nation, was back in England lobbying the Queen and the War Office to set up a Royal Commission to inquire into sanitary conditions in hospitals and barracks and the administration of the Army Medical Department. She had no hesitation in assuming a monopoly of compassion for the troops, and by now she was quite literally a power behind the throne.

Barry, too, had returned home on leave that year. For the first time in her army career she was without a friend in high office. Since Raglan's death she could command no influence at army headquarters – with painfully predictable results. She was barely a month in town when news arrived of her next posting: she was to be shunted off to Canada after serving for more than forty years in the tropics.

She wrote laconically of the transfer to a colleague:

So I am to go to Canada to cool off myself after such a long residence in the Tropics and hot countries. You are to go to Dublin, which is to be a 3 year station and who goes to Corfu is not yet known. This much for changes and chances in this world of woe and this vale of tears as scholars say.

The arrangements were made by our Deputy Inspector of Hospitals – no doubt for your wellfare!

Barry might have sounded philosophical but at heart she was

unhappy and worried. Did she suspect that Florence Nightingale, who now held enormous influence at the Army Medical Department, wanted her out of the way?

Her leave, at any rate, was the shortest of her career. She spent the remainder of it at Lowther Castle, the home of the Earl of Lonsdale, who had once played host to Lord Charles Somerset. The vast, pseudo-Gothic castle, with its fine deer park, held a room for every day of the year. Lord Lonsdale, a splendid eccentric, enjoyed entertaining and Scott, Wordsworth and most of the leading literary and artistic figures of the day had been his guests. None of them attracted more attention in the town than Dr James Barry, driving in Miss Lonsdale's carriage with her own black servant in attendance.

Over the years, the gossip about Barry remained fairly consistent. She was renowned for her 'caustic waspish temper', her tiny hands, almost ashen countenance and pinched, aquiline features, set off by an unmistakable flaxen wig (in earlier stories it had been a reddish wig). If one is to believe the gossips who met her in the fifties (and wrote about her forty years later), everyone knew 'he' was a woman.

Canada, however, was certainly no place for a woman – let alone a woman who had spent two-thirds of her life in hot climates. Now, for the first time she was to be exposed to the rigours of a Canadian winter. When she arrived the thermometer was several degrees below zero. Despite her frail frame, she proved indomitable, refusing to let the icy weather prevent her from going about her work with her usual energy. From her handsome, pillared house in an elegant district of Montreal she would emerge, muffled up in musk-ox furs but immaculately dressed with 'a long silk bow on the breast of her uniform frock coat, dandified boots of patent leather and long fingered white gloves'.

The year that Barry arrived the first club in Canada for gentlemen opened, the St James Club in Montreal, modelled on its namesake in London. A very decorous and gentlemanly establishment, the club prided itself on good food (partridge and champagne appeared on the menu every night) and good manners. The servants who waited at table were ordered to 'show attention to their general appearance and to avoid loud talking and other disagreeable noises'. Members were banned from playing pool in the billiards room and on Sunday even billiards was frowned upon.

For the new industrialists and the bankers who were growing in importance with the thriving little town, the Club became a second home. Since Montreal was a garrison town, a number of the officers stationed there were granted the privilege of becoming full members although they remained ineligible to serve on the committee. Barry was among the first to be invited to take up a subscription. When she entered that inviolably masculine atmosphere, she must have been struck by the irony of the situation. But perhaps, after forty years' service in the Army, she felt more at home in the billiards room than in the boudoir. Certainly her interests and her talk belonged to a man's world. A legend exists to this day that she fought a duel in Canada, but that seems too absurd to contemplate – even for Barry. And at her age she could hardly feign flirtations with pretty girls or cavort around the ballroom as she had done in her prime. Her swaggering appearance in full-dress uniform with sword and spurs did, however, still cause a stir when she turned up on Sundays to attend services at Christchurch Cathedral. And her temper evidently was not improved by the climate.

The only practical form of transport was the sleigh and it was a precarious and often painful means of travel. As it bounced and slithered in the ruts of the icy road, Barry was frequently flung on the floor and she could be heard cursing her wretched footmen 'in a voice like the squall of angry seagull'. But she liked to travel fast, even though she was frightened and bitterly cold, as she sat wrapped up in her furs only six inches from the ground. Her horses were frequently half buried in the snow and sometimes the bright red sleigh overturned completely. Nevertheless she journeyed hundreds of miles to Quebec, Kingston and Toronto to visit the men and the barracks and report on their condition.

On her visits she concerned herself with the everyday details of the soldiers' life. She suggested modernizing the barracks by introducing water pipes instead of relying on wells that froze up every winter and expressed strong criticism of the sewage and drainage systems throughout the Command.

Perhaps the most remarkable quality that Barry brought to

dull routine work was her imagination. In Quebec, for example, she noted that the barracks had no oven and soldiers were subjected to an endless diet of boiled beef. She recommended 'the cheering change of a roast'.

In Canada, as in every station where she had served, she was concerned about widespread drunkenness among the troops. It was a familiar story. 'The Commanding Officers are indefatigable in their efforts to suppress intemperance', she wrote, 'but the cheapness of liquor and the general tendency of the soldiers to drink ... baffles their efforts.' Instead of dismissing the soldiers as drunk and irresponsible, however, she saw the problem from their point of view:

Probably one of the causes and a great one is the absence of separate accommodation for married persons as, however limited, a room for each family would indeed be not only a great boon to the soldier, but diminish intemperance, which is the chief cause of crime, punishment, sickness and death. This I annually iterated and reiterated.

(One can almost hear the authorities sighing in exasperation.)

In this report, as in many others she wrote, her humanity breaks through:

For example, a woman humbly born but modestly and religiously educated is suddenly placed in a Barrack room with ten or twenty men, perhaps some married. She becomes frightened and disgusted, next becomes habituated and in despair has recourse to drunkenness and not infrequently her husband, a good man, joins with his wife and becomes the occupant of a cell in a military prison.

If only, wrote Barry, a similar room had been provided for each married couple 'they might live with decency and bring up their children in the fear of God without being tainted with the awful and disgusting language of a Barrack Room'.

Despite the romantic legend that surrounds Barry, her work was essentially practical. She wrote to the Deputy Quartermaster General in August 1858 requesting urgently 'that hair mattresses and hair or feather pillows be substituted for the paliasses and straw pillows now issued to the Hospitals in this Command, as it must be evident the great comfort it would be to a poor sufferer to rest his emaciated and feverish limbs on something more genial than hard straw'. And she begged that if there were not enough material in the Command, application home should be made immediately.

Yet despite her concern for the soldiers' comfort, she did not believe in mollycoddling the men. She was satisfied that in Canada the troops were reasonably healthy and wanted to see them active too: 'From a sanitary point of view nothing can be more desirable to the general health of a soldier than employment and when possible in the open air.'

But she wanted more than that. She asked for libraries with a good selection of books for the troops and suggested that athletics should be encouraged. She was, in fact, pleading for a civilized soldiery – something hitherto considered impossible. She wanted to help to put an end to the traditional view of the British soldier as 'the scum of the earth'. But to push her reforms through she first had to convince army officers who still bought and sold their commissions and cared very little for the lives and interests of their men. It must have been a hard and dispiriting grind but Barry did not spare herself. By April of 1859 it was clear that the overwork and the extremes of a cold climate had taken their toll.

On the 20th of April 1859 the minute book of the St James Club records that 'The Committee submits a letter received from Dr Barry, Inspector General of Hospitals, stating that being unable, from ill-health, to enjoy the privileges of the Club he wishes his name to be withdrawn from the list of Members.' The Committee resolved to accept Barry's resignation, but to place her name 'on the list of supernumerary members'. (This meant that she could resume her membership by paying the yearly subscription without any formalities.)

The doctor who attended her during her illness, Dr G. W. Campbell, later became Dean of the McGill Medical School. As he used to tell his students,

> If I had not stood in some awe of Inspector General Barry's rank and medical attainments, I would have examined him – that is, her – far more thoroughly. Because I did not and because his – confound it, her – bedroom was always in almost total darkness when I paid my calls, this, ah, crucial point escaped me.

That year an epidemic of influenza swept Canada. Barry caught the flu and bronchitis so badly that on the 14th of May

1859, weak and exhausted she had to come home. She boarded a steamship at Quebec bound for Liverpool. The sea journey upset her as all sea journeys did, and by the time she arrived home, on the 26th May, she was so ill that she was obliged to stay up north for a few days before risking the arduous journey to London.

On her own admission, Barry looked 'unusually delicate and meagre' when she reached London and 'within three days scarcely recovered from the sea sickness during a rough and tempestuous voyage' she was ordered before a medical board.

To her obvious disgust the doctors required to report on her health were junior to her: 'perfect strangers to me and to my peculiar habits'. She heard nothing from them until the 19th of July when she was placed on half-pay. Because of her illness she had not completed her period of service as Inspector General and she was bitterly disappointed at a retirement which despite her age and state of health she regarded as premature. She once again sat down and penned a five-page 'Memorandum of Services'. She begged to be sent back to Canada where she had only twenty more months to serve which would have saved her 'great pecuniary loss'. She pointed out that she had only once taken leave of absence on private affairs and 'then only when I conceived my prospects in the service were seriously compromised for want of a personal appeal at Head Quarters'.

Each change of station, she explained, subjected her to an 'immense personal outlay' because the climates of each posting varied so much. Every time she moved it 'entailed a sacrifice of property'.

She closed the memorandum rather wistfully: 'I am now prepared to serve Her Majesty in any quarter of the Globe to which I may be sent and am loath to close a career which impartially may be deemed to have been a useful and faithful one without some special mark of Her Majesty's gracious favour.' Did she hope for an honour?

She received nothing. A month after her memorandum begging for reinstatement reached the War Office, Sir Andrew Smith, the Director General of the Army Medical Department, died. (He had been up at Edinburgh with Barry during her student days and served in South Africa with her and she might reasonably have considered herself a suitable successor. The Army was seriously short of senior medical officers.) But once again her talent for making enemies stood in her way. 'It seems', wrote the omnipresent Miss Nightingale, 'as if there was not one man in the Department whom one wished to see Director General.'

Barry was, perhaps, unsuited for the post of Director General of the Army Medical Department. Even as a young officer she had an unfortunate tendency to display an independent mind and bypass the 'usual channels', thus causing trouble; and even from her own point of view it might have been undesirable to be so much in the public eye with the inevitable risk of discovery that that would bring. It is not at all clear whether there was any officer left alive who knew her secret, although Florence Nightingale's letter, written after Barry's death, suggests that there was gossip at the Horse Guards. But even if she could not serve as Director General it seems incredible that with competent senior medical officers so scarce, no use could be made of her talents.

So far as the Army Medical Department was concerned she was retired and useless. If she grew bitter and querulous, it is hardly surprising. She had spent all her life fighting for better living conditions for the lower orders – not only for the troops, but for lepers and lunatics, blacks and convicts. Long before the Crimean War she had written report after report about the need to improve hospitals and barracks, and the diet and leisure of the ordinary soldier. As for hygiene, she had urged the need for rigorous cleanliness more than forty years earlier.

Yet it was Miss Nightingale who won the honour and fame. Now Barry had to face the reality that she was redundant and alone, an ex-army doctor who could never relax her disguise. In her time she had seen the fashionable world of the Regency give way inexorably to the prim and prosperous Victorian era. The pace of life had quickened beyond recognition. Railways and steamships and the new macadamized roads had transformed travel and communications. Slavery had been abolished, but in the thriving industrial towns of the Midlands men, women and children worked in conditions that rivalled anything the Colonies had to offer. Life had grown more complex, more organized and more impersonal – and it was passing Barry by.

In her retirement she travelled to the places where she had been useful, where she had been known. One gets the feeling that she was desperately trying to escape. In 1860 she visited Jamaica and made friends with the manager of a local drug store in Kingston, a Mr McCrindle and his family. They often exchanged visits. Although a strict vegetarian, Barry kept a 'well-set table' for her friends and when she wanted a haircut she would drive to the family house (above the store), send for a barber and get her hair cut in the drawing-room. Perhaps all those stories about a wig were merely malicious?

J. C. McCrindle, the son of Barry's friends, wrote to the *Glasgow Herald* about her in 1949, when he himself was a very old man. Barry, it seems, fell ill in Jamaica and sent for his father. She then, so the story goes, showed him a small black box and asked him to promise that, in the event of her death, he would 'get the box and keep it until it was sent for...'

A few months later when Mrs McCrindle gave birth to a daughter, Barry gave the infant a solid silver drinking mug, a silver knife, fork and a spoon, all engraved 'Presented by Dr James Barry, Inspector General of Hospitals in the West Indies'. She wanted to adopt the baby, Mr McCrindle recalled, and said she would send her to a cousin in Scotland – 'I think a Lady Jane Grey or Gordon...' Again the mystery. Was Barry romancing or Mr McCrindle? Or was there a Scottish connection?

Some exaggeration has undoubtedly crept in. According to Mr McCrindle, Dr Barry told his parents she had fought a duel and *killed* an opponent in South Africa! But she did leave the McCrindles two solid souvenirs, besides the baby's presents: a signet ring with a crest on it, and a ring with 'Sacred to the memory of Marion' engraved inside. Was Marion perhaps Barry's own name before she became 'James'? Or did the ring belong to Mrs Bulkley – *Mary Anne* Bulkley?

Long after her death, Barry evoked memories and stories. Her life was lived among Generals and Colonels, sharing their jokes (if not their after-dinner port), and in every situation where she served she was almost certainly the subject of an after-dinner anecdote herself.

Colonel Rogers, the enterprising author of *The Modern*

Sphinx, recalled travelling with this 'remarkable character' aboard a ship plying between St Thomas and Barbados. Rogers (who was only a Captain in those days) occupied the same cabin.

I in the top, she in the lower berth – of course without any suspicion of her sex on my part. I well remember how in a harsh and peevish voice she ordered me out of the cabin – blow high, blow low – while she dressed in the morning. 'Now then youngster, clear out of my cabin while I dress' she would say.

By the winter of 1864 Barry was back in England and again a guest of the Earl of Lonsdale; 'The attenuated form of the lady was generally understood to be due to a vegetarian diet and many were the jokes that were passed at "The Doctor's" expense during her ladyship's sojourn at the Castle.'

From Cumberland she returned to London and the end of her travels. She took lodgings in a dentist's house in Marylebone. By now she must have felt that the purpose of her existence had gone and when an 'epidemic of summer diarrhoea' spread through the borough Barry, who had nursed patients with the disease back to health all over the world, neglected her own diet. By mid-July she was ill – for only the third time in her life. Despite the ministrations of Staff Surgeon McKinnon, she soon weakened. At four in the morning on the 25th of July 1865, Dr James Barry died. (It was, curiously enough, the anniversary of the day, thirty-nine years earlier, when she had performed the spectacular Caesarian operation that had saved her godson, James Barry Munnik.)

An intriguing story exists that two footmen in gorgeous livery called at the lodgings in Margaret Street and removed all her belongings – including her little poodle (the last of the Psyches), her diamond ring and the mysterious black box. Her Negro servant apparently went back to Jamaica, his passage paid by an unknown benefactor.

Barry herself was buried in what was then a prominent position in Kensal Green Cemetery. The plot cost three guineas. But a mystery still surrounds the identity of the patron who so carefully removed all trace of her masquerade.

The most likely assumption is that it was the Beauforts. But no firm evidence has come to light and the present Duke of

Beaufort disclaims all knowledge of his family's connection with the doctor.

Barry's story, so tantalizingly incomplete, did not end with her death. After the revelations of the charwoman, Sophia Bishop, the speculation which had been held in check during her lifetime grew wilder. It took two forms. On the one hand she was depicted as a detestable freak. An unknown officer of the Buffs painted a portrait in oils of her in dress uniform with a monkey's face.

On the other hand novelists and playwrights were not slow to exploit the romantic possibilities of her career.

In *Dr James Barry – her secret life*, by Jessica Grove and Olga Racster, Barry is portrayed as a passionate young woman who suppresses her love (which in their version of the story is for Captain Cloete, the man with whom, in reality, she fought a duel). The novel is in diary form:

> 'Captain Cloete, sir,' I said. 'Don't forget what I say. Keep hold of love. It is the most precious thing the world has to offer. Good-bye.' I held out my hand, but he refused it, bowed instead and went out.
>
> The spirit of youth seemed to pass from my life as I listened to the footsteps of Cloete and Lavinia on the flagged path which led to the gate. When it closed it was as though all the joyousness the world could offer had been shut out of my heart. The gulf between myself and normal life suddenly widened into a mighty chasm into which I did not care whether I fell or not.
>
> Oh Cloete, Cloete . . . I never realised till now what you meant to me . . . I told you love was the one precious thing in life . . . More than ever do I know it, now that you are lost to me!

For the next half century Barry's amazing life was explained in terms which concentrate on an imaginary motive for her masquerade – the love of an officer. Needless to say this sentimental treatment managed to obscure her real achievements as a doctor and a social reformer. Even on the plaque outside the Barry Ward (the 10th Ward for Female Officers) in the Queen Alexandra Military Hospital, her vocation is attributed to a misleading cause and the details of her career are inaccurately recorded.

James Barry entered the Army in 1813 as a Hospital Assistant to become successively, Assistant Surgeon, Surgeon Major, Deputy Inspector and finally Inspector General in 1858.

Lord Albemarle, who met Barry when the latter was Staff Surgeon to the Governor of the Cape of Good Hope, wrote this description of her: 'most skilful of physicians and most wayward of men. In appearance a beardless lad with an unmistakable Scotch type of countenance, with reddish hair and high cheekbones. There was a certain effeminacy in his manner which he was always striving to overcome.'

Inspector General Barry died suddenly in his sleep aged 71. A post-mortem examination revealed him to be a woman. Bit by bit the story leaked out – a 16-year-old Scottish girl who loved a junior doctor suddenly ordered out to Wellington's Army in Spain. There were no women nurses in those days so to join the Army James Barry had to pass herself off as a man and go as a medical assistant to the Army.

Despite Isobel Rae's sterling vindication of Barry in 1958, the first factual biography ever written, modern attempts to discredit her persist.

Professor Kirby, a musicologist who interested himself for years in the problem of Barry's sex wrote numerous articles in South African medical journals designed to prove that she could not have been a woman. In his writings, he brings a considerable weight of medical learning to bear on the subject of hermaphroditism, but never succeeds in establishing that Barry was indeed a hermaphrodite. His obsession with the specifically sexual identity is typical of a common – and predominantly male – assumption that a woman by nature would have been incapable of sustaining the masquerade and attaining such professional prominence.

Today, perhaps, her adventure seems more credible. Women do become doctors and even serve in armies on equal terms with men. What makes Barry so exceptional is that she anticipated feminine emancipation by nearly a hundred years. And she did so not as a woman but from within the stiff conventions of an exclusively male world. It is a tribute to her courage that she managed to subordinate her private life to her professional work yet survived as a human being. And never in her forty-six years' service in the Army did she betray her ideals as a doctor or as a 'perfect gentleman'.

Postscript

In writing this book I collected all the documents about Dr Barry that I could find and structured the narrative from them.

The Muniment Room of the Royal Army Medical Corps, London, houses the Barry Papers, the most important records. (Isobel Rae, Barry's first factual biographer, discovered most of them. I added my own finds to the collection: the Barry/Bulkley letters, parish records of the Barry family from Cork, the Proceedings of the Court Martial at St Helena, letters from Malta, etc.)

The Public Record Office has the fullest documentation of her career. (Barry's 'Statement of Home and Foreign Services' (WO:25/3899) is a useful starting point for research.) My other sources include the British Museum, the Scottish National Library, the Manuscript Room of Edinburgh University Library, the Ogilvie Trust and the National Army Museum, the Library of the Royal Commonwealth Society, and the Wellcome Library.

In the brief bibliography below I have included only those books that bear directly on the life of Dr Barry or her extended family.

Albemarle, 6th Earl of. *Fifty Years of My Life*. London 1876.
Some barbed and often quoted passages about Barry occur in this book written almost fifty years after their meeting in Cape Town.

Buchan, Earl of. *Anonymous and Fugitive Essays*. Edinburgh

1812. These essays, written under the pen name 'Albanicus' reflect the author's remarkably advanced views on the education of women.

Burke, E. *The Correspondence of Edmund Burke,* Volumes I–III. Cambridge University Press, London, 1958–61. Burke's letters reveal the extent of his generous patronage of James Barry, R.A., and his concern for John Barry, the artist's father. They also illustrate something of his standing with the blue-stockings, and with Mrs Boscawen in particular.

Dillon, Sir William Henry. *A Narrative of My Professional Adventures.* Printed for the Navy Records Society, 1856. This book, published during Barry's lifetime, establishes the fact that some contemporaries at least, guessed her sex.

Fenton, J. *Journal of Mrs Fenton.* London 1901. The author, who stayed on Mauritius in 1828 when Barry was stationed there, narrates her impressions of the doctor.

Fryer, Dr Edward. *The Works of James Barry, R.A.* London 1809. This book, a result of the collaboration between General Miranda, Lord Buchan and Dr Fryer, provides evidence of the artist's close association with Edmund Burke and Lord Buchan.

Laidler, P. and Gelfand, M. *South Africa, its Medical History 1652–1898.* Cape Town 1971. In this comprehensive history, two carefully documented chapters are devoted almost exclusively to Barry.

Las Casas, Comte de. *Journal of the Private Life and Conversations of Napoleon at St Helena.* London 1823. Las Casas' impressions of the young Dr Barry at the Cape.

Millar, Anthony Kendal. *Plantagenet in South Africa.* London 1965. Somewhat indulgent biography of the life and times of Barry's friend Lord Charles Somerset. This book was strongly recommended to the author by the present Duchess of Beaufort and the Beaufort family historian, Mrs Horatia Durrant.

Miranda, F. *Archivo Del General Miranda.* Caracas and Havana 1929–50. Volumes 16–18. These archives (housed in the British Museum) present the most interesting and incomplete evidence of Dr Barry's origins.

Rae, Isobel. *The Strange Story of Dr James Barry.* London

1958. Painstaking biography which brought the Barry papers to light and presented new factual evidence.

Theal, G. M. *Records of the Cape Colony*. London 1903. Volumes 15–33 contain the official records of Barry's career in South Africa, including reports, correspondence, etc.

Inevitably my quest for Dr Barry involved me in lengthy correspondence and dealings with people all over the world. I am grateful to all those who have helped me. In particular I would like to thank: Major-General Alastair MacLennan, Curator of the R.A.M.C. Museum for his sympathetic assistance throughout; Mrs Treleaven (formerly Mrs James Barry Munnik) for allowing me access to old family documents and newspaper cuttings. Professor William L. Pressly of the Department of History of Art at Yale University for generously sending me copies of letters from Mrs Bulkley to her brother; Dr Thelma Gutsche and Anthony Kendal Millar and his wife for their helpful references from South Africa.

I am also indebted to Lotte Lowenthal, who spent months working at the Public Record Office and discovered the Barry letters from Malta; to Mr T. H. Bullock of Bristol for tracing the Beaufort connection with Stoke Park; to Mrs Thena Kendal for reading the manuscript and making some valuable suggestions; to Barbara Phillips and Elizabeth Radice for typing the manuscript with care and enthusiasm, and not least to my two editors, Edward Bennett and Elaine Hopton for their advice and encouragement.

Index

Compiled by Susan Kennedy